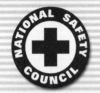 **National Safety Council** ®

Bloodborne Pathogens

Fourth Edition

Karen Carruthers, R.N.
Senior Technical Writer
Exactis.com
Denver, CO

Mark Jackson, M.D.
Director of Student Health Services
Cutler Health Center
University of Maine
Orono, ME

Sally McKinnon, B.S.N.
Associate for Clinical Management
Cutler Health Center
University of Maine
Orono, ME

JONES AND BARTLETT PUBLISHERS

Sudbury, Massachusetts

BOSTON   TORONTO   LONDON   SINGAPORE

Jones and Bartlett Publishers
40 Tall Pine Drive, Sudbury, MA 01776
508-443-5000
800-832-0034
nsc@jbpub.com
www.nsc.jbpub.com

Jones and Bartlett Publishers Canada
2406 Nikanna Road
Mississauga, ON L5C 2W6
CANADA

Jones and Bartlett Publishers International
Barb House, Barb Mews
London W6 7PA
UK

 National Safety Council®
Emergency Care Programs
1121 Spring Lake Drive
Itasca, IL 60143-3201
(630) 285-1121
(800) 621-6244
www.nsc.org

Executive Director, Home & Community Safety and Health Group: Donna Siegfried

Program Development & Training Manager, Home & Community Safety and Health Group: Barbara Caracci

Production Credits
Chief Executive Officer: Clayton E. Jones
Chief Operating Officer: Donald W. Jones, Jr.
Executive V.P. and Publisher: Tom Manning
V.P. and Managing Editor: Judith H. Hauck
V.P., Sales and Marketing: Paul Shepardson
V.P., Production and Design: Anne Spencer
V.P., Manufacturing and Inventory Control: Therese Bräuer
Publisher, EMS & Aquatics: Lawrence D. Newell
Emergency Care Senior Acquisitions Editor: Tracy Foss
Director of Marketing, EMS and Health Sciences: Kimberly Brophy
Emergency Care Associate Editor: Jennifer Reed

Production Editor: Linda S. DeBruyn
Interactive Technology Director: W. Scott Smith
Design and Composition: Studio Montage
Illustrations: Rolin Graphics
Interior Photos: Richard Nye
Cover Design: Studio Montage
Cover Photographs (clockwise from top left):
  Digital Imagery © 2000 PhotoDisc, Inc.; Maryland Institute of Emergency Medical Services System (MIEMMS); Steve Ferry, P&P Communications; © Yoav Levy/Phototake/PictureQuest
Printing and Binding: Courier Company

The information presented in this book is based on the most recent recommendations of responsible medical/industrial sources. The National Safety Council, the author and the publisher, however, make no guarantee as to, and assume no responsibility for, correctness, sufficiency or completeness of such information or recommendations. Other or additional safety measures may be required under particular circumstances.

The OSHA Bloodborne Pathogens Standard is an evolving standard. The authors are in no way responsible for changes made in the standard after the printing of this text. Annual training is required to keep up with changes in the standard.

Library of Congress Cataloging-in-Publication Data
Bloodborne pathogens /National Safety Council.–4th ed.
                p.   cm.
        Previous editions published under title.
        Includes index.
        ISBN 0-7637-1317-1 (alk. paper)
        1.Bloodborne infections–Prevention.
        I. National Safety Council.   II. Title.
        RA642.B56 T48 2000
        614.4–dc21   00-049735

Printed in the United States of America
05 04 03 02   10 9 8 7 6 5 4 3

About the National Safety Council Program

Congratulations on selecting the National Safety Council's First Aid and CPR program! You join good company, as the National Safety Council has successfully trained over 6 million people worldwide in first aid and cardiopulmonary resuscitation (CPR). The National Safety Council's training network of nearly 10,000 instructors at over 4,000 sites worldwide has established the National Safety Council programs as the standard by which all others are judged.

In setting the standards, the National Safety Council has worked in close cooperation with hundreds of national and international organizations, thousands of corporations, thousands of leading educators, dozens of leading medical organizations, and hundreds of state and local governmental agencies. Their collective input has helped create programs that stand alone in quality. Consider just a few of the National Safety Council's current collaborations:

World's Leading Medical Organizations

The National Safety Council is currently working with both the American Academy of Orthopedic Surgeons (AAOS), Wilderness Medical Society (WMS), and the American Heart Association to help bring innovative, new training programs to the marketplace. The National Safety Council and the AAOS are developing a new First Responder program and the National Safety Council and the WMS are developing the first-of-its-kind wilderness first aid program.

Spanning the Globe

Across the globe, from Boston to Bangkok, from Miami to Milan, from Seattle to Stockholm, people are trained with National Safety Council programs. National Safety Council first aid and CPR programs are already used in your area.

World's Leading Corporations

Thousands of corporations including Westinghouse, Exxon, General Motors, Ameritech, and U.S. West have selected many of the National Safety Council emergency care programs to train employees.

World's Leading Colleges and Universities

Hundreds of leading colleges and universities are working closely with the National Safety Council to fully develop and implement the Internet Initiative that will establish the National Safety Council as the leading online provider of emergency care programs.

Most importantly, in selecting the National Safety Council programs, you can feel confident that the programs are of the highest quality. You can rely on the National Safety Council. Founded in 1913, the National Safety Council is dedicated to protecting life, promoting health, and reducing accidental death. For nearly 90 years, the National Safety Council has been the world's leading authority on safety/injury education.

National Safety Council ®

Table of Contents

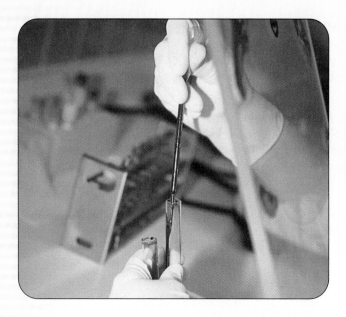

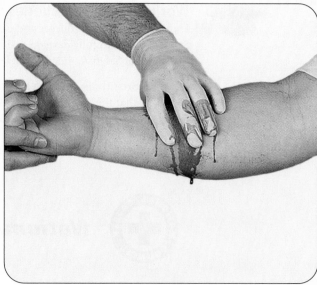

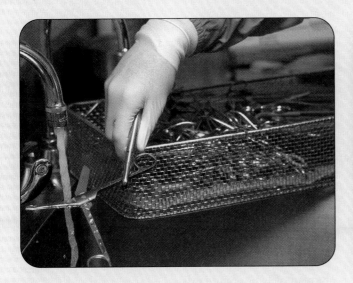

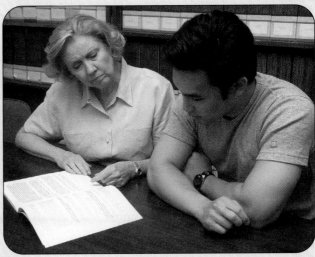

Acknowledgments

Principal Reviewers

We wish to thank the following individuals and companies for their contributions to the various editions of this manual.

Peggy Baum
Health and Safety Administrator
University of Maine
Orono, ME

Carol Bufton
Minnesota Safety Council
St. Paul, MN

Richard Cooper
SEMTA
Rye, NH

Kay Farrell
Safety and Health Council of Greater Omaha
Omaha, NE

First Aid and CPR Advisory Committee
New Jersey State Safety Council
Cranford, NJ

Donna Gates
Health Care and Nursing Consultants
Lexington, KY

David A. Gibbs
Safety Compliance Specialist
State of Maine
Bureau of Labor Standards
Augusta, Maine

Lynne Lamstein, M.S.I.H.
Occupational Health Specialist
State of Maine
Department of Labor
Bureau of Labor Standards
Augusta, Maine

Safety Council of Maryland
Baltimore, MD

Jose Salazar
Loudoun County Fire and Rescue
Leesburg, Virginia

Donna Siegfried
First Aid Institute
National Safety Council
Itasca, Illinois

Alton Thygerson, Ph.D.
Brigham Young University
Provo, Utah

Chapter 1

Introduction

Overview

Since 1992, employer implementation of the OSHA Bloodborne Pathogens Standard has been continually guided by OSHA's interpretation of the Standard, OSHA's citations for violations of the Standard and court rulings specific to the Standard. Training about the risks and hazards associated with tasks involving blood and Other Potentially Infectious Materials (OPIM) has improved employee safety. The Standard has motivated manufacturers to introduce new engineering controls (e.g., needleless systems) and develop and produce a wide variety of products that offer greater choice for worksite safety and personal protection.

Despite the advances in engineering work practices, and personal protective equipment, the health risks posed by the handling of blood and OPIM remain very high. The requirements of the OSHA Bloodborne Pathogens Standard continue to be essential in maintaining safe work environments for all employees engaged in handling blood and OPIM.

Throughout this manual you will see references to California OSHA (CalOSHA). These notations are clearly marked with a symbol to indicate that this interpretation of the standard is taken from the CalOSHA standard. CalOSHA has been referenced in cases where their interpretation of the Standard was more stringent than Federal OSHA, or where it was felt that their interpretation or requirements could benefit others. Regardless, these notations are clearly marked so you will be able to distinguish between the requirements of the Federal Standard and the CalOSHA Standard.

The Standard requires that you learn the content of the Bloodborne Pathogens Standard; that you receive training on the categories defined within the Standard; and that you receive site-specific training to properly implement the requirements in your work environment. This unit provides an overview of the OSHA Bloodborne Pathogens Standard.

OSHA Bloodborne Pathogens Standard

OSHA Bloodborne Pathogens Regulations Section 1910.1030

Part 1910-[Amended]

Subpart Z-[Amended]

1. The general authority citation for subpart Z of 29 CFR part 1910 continues to read as follows and a new citation for 1910.1030 is added:

Authority: Secs. 6 and 8, Occupational Safety and Health Act, 29 U.S.C. 655, 657, Secretary of Labor's Orders Nos. 12-71 (36 CFR 8754), 8-76 (41 CFR 25059), or 9-83 (48 CFR 35736), as applicable; and 29 CFR part 1911.
*   *   *   *   *

Section 1910.1030 also issued under 29 U.S.C. 853.

2. Section 1910.1030 is added to read as follows:

1910.1030 Bloodborne Pathogens.

(a) Scope and Application

This section applies to all occupational exposure to blood or other potentially infectious materials as defined by paragraph (b) of this section.

(b) Definitions

For purposes of this section, the following shall apply:

Assistant Secretary means the Assistant Secretary of Labor for Occupational Safety and Health, or designated representative.

Blood means human blood, human blood components, and products made from human blood.

Bloodborne Pathogens means pathogenic microorganisms that are present in human blood and can cause disease in humans. These pathogens include, but are not limited to, Hepatitis B Virus [HBV] and Human Immunodeficiency Virus [HIV].

Clinical Laboratory means a workplace where diagnostic or other screening procedures are performed on blood or other potentially infectious materials.

Contaminated means the presence or the reasonably anticipated presence of blood or other potentially infectious materials on an item or surface.

Contaminated Laundry means laundry which has been soiled with blood or other potentially infectious materials or may contain sharps.

Contaminated Sharps means any contaminated object that can penetrate the skin including, but not limited to, needles, scalpels, broken glass, broken capillary tubes, and exposed ends of dental wires.

Decontamination means the use of physical or chemical means to remove, inactivate, or destroy bloodborne pathogens on a surface or item to the point where they are no longer capable of transmitting infectious particles and the surface or item is rendered safe for handling, use, or disposal.

Director means the Director of the National Institute for Occupational Safety and Health, U.S. Department of Health and Human Services, or designated representative.

Engineering Controls means controls (e.g., sharps disposal containers, self-sheathing needles) that isolate or remove the bloodborne pathogens hazard from the workplace.

Exposure Incident means a specific eye, mouth, other mucous membrane, non-intact skin, or parenteral contact with blood or other potentially infectious materials that results from the performance of an employee's duties.

Handwashing Facilities means a facility providing an adequate supply of running potable water, soap, and single use towels or hot air drying machines.

Licensed Health Care Professional is a person whose legally permitted scope of practice allows him or her to independently perform the activities required by paragraph (f) Hepatitis B vaccination and Post-Exposure Evaluation and Follow-Up.

HBV means Hepatitis B Virus.

HIV means Human Immunodeficiency Virus.

Occupational Exposure means reasonably anticipated skin, eye, mucous membrane, or parenteral contact with blood or other potentially infectious materials that may result from the performance of an employee's duties.

Other Potentially Infectious Materials means

(1) The following human body fluids: semen, vaginal secretions, cerebrospinal fluid, synovial fluid, pleural fluid, pericardial fluid, peritoneal fluid, amniotic fluid, saliva in dental procedures, any body fluid that is visibly contaminated with blood, and all body fluids in situations where it is difficult or impossible to differentiate between body fluids;

(2) Any unfixed tissue or organ (other than intact skin) from a human (living or dead); and

(3) HIV-containing cell or tissue cultures, organ cultures, and HIV- or HBV-containing culture medium or other solutions; and blood, organs, or other tissues from experimental animals infected with HIV or HBV.

Parenteral means piercing mucous membranes or the skin barrier through such events as needlesticks, human bites, cuts, and abrasions.

Figure 1-1   OSHA Bloodborne Pathogen Standard

What Is the OSHA Bloodborne Pathogens Standard?

In 1991, OSHA (Occupational Safety and Health Administration) issued its final regulation on occupational exposure to bloodborne pathogens (29 CFR 1910.1030). OSHA determined that employees face a significant health risk as the result of occupational exposure to blood and other potentially infectious materials (OPIM) because they may contain bloodborne pathogens. This standard provides requirements for employers to follow to ensure employee safety with regard to occupational exposure to bloodborne pathogens. **▲ Figure 1-1**

Bloodborne pathogens include, but are not limited to, hepatitis B virus (HBV), which causes hepatitis B; human immunodeficiency virus (HIV), which causes acquired immunodeficiency syndrome (AIDS); hepatitis C virus (HCV); human T-lymphotrophic virus Type 1; and the pathogens which cause diseases such as malaria, syphilis, arboviral infections, relapsing fever, and viral hemorrhagic fever.

Hazards from bloodborne pathogens can be minimized or eliminated by using a combination of engineering and work practice controls, personal protective clothing and equipment, training, medical surveillance, hepatitis B vaccination and signs and labels. Both the Standard and CPL 2-2.44C became effective on March 6, 1992. CPL 2-2.44D became effective November 5, 1999 and cancelled CPL 2-2.44C.

This edition of the National Safety Council Bloodborne Pathogens manual continues to provide guidance specific to 29 CFR 1910.1030 and incorporates clarifications found in CPL 2-2.44D, OSHA interpretations, and OSHA citations.

Who Needs OSHA BBP Training?

The scope of the Standard is not limited to employees with job classifications that may that have occupational exposure to blood and other potentially infectious materials. In the case of a warehouse employee trained in first aid and identified by the employer as responsible for rendering medical assistance as part of his/her job duties, that employee is covered by the standard.

The Standard includes the potential for exposure, not just actual exposure. For example, a front desk receptionist may not have an actual exposure to a bleeding patient, but the potential for exposure may exist.

Employees

Any employee who has occupational exposure to blood or other potentially infectious material is included within the scope of the Standard. This includes part-time, temporary, healthcare workers known as "per diem" employees and volunteers.

OSHA jurisdiction extends only to private business employees in the workplace. It does not extend to students if they are not considered employees, to state, county, or municipal employees, to health care professionals who are sole practitioners or partners, and to the self-employed.

Any employee who has potential for occupational exposure to blood or OPIM is required to receive training according to the bloodborne pathogens standard. The following job classifications may be associated with tasks that have occupational exposure to blood or OPIM, but the standard is not limited to employees in these positions. **▶ Figure 1-2**

· Physicians, physician's assistants, nurses, nurse practitioners, and other healthcare employees in clinics and physicians' offices

· Employees of clinical and diagnostic laboratories

· Housekeepers in healthcare and other facilities

- Personnel in hospital laundries or commercial laundries that service healthcare or public safety institutions

- Tissue bank personnel

- Employees in blood banks and plasma centers who collect, transport, and test blood

- Freestanding clinic employees (e.g., hemodialysis clinics, urgent care clinics, health maintenance organization (HMO) clinics, and family planning clinics)

- Employees in clinics in industrial, educational, and correctional facilities (e.g., those who collect blood, and clean and dress wounds)

- Employees designated to provide emergency first aid

- Dentists, dental hygienists, dental assistants and dental laboratory technicians

- Staff of institutions for the developmentally disabled

- Hospice employees

- Home healthcare workers

- Staff of nursing homes and long-term care facilities

- Employees of funeral homes and mortuaries

- HIV and HBV research laboratory and production facility workers

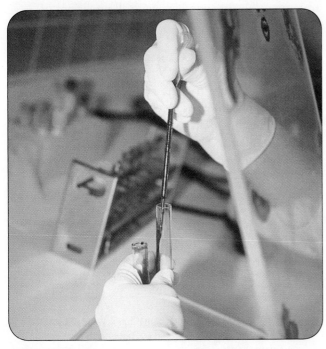

Figure 1-2   All procedures should be performed to minimize splashing.

- Employees handling regulated waste; custodial workers required to clean up contaminated sharps or spills of blood or OPIM

- Medical equipment service and repair personnel

- Emergency medical technicians, paramedics, and other emergency medical service providers

- Fire fighters, law enforcement personnel, and correctional officers

- Maintenance workers, such as plumbers, in healthcare facilities and employees of substance abuse clinics

Employers and Employment Agencies

An employment agency refers job applicants to potential employers but does not put these workers on the payroll or otherwise establish an employment relationship with them; thus, the employment agency is not the employer of these workers. The company that uses these workers, e.g., a hospital, is the employer of these workers and is responsible for providing training according to the Bloodborne Pathogens Standard.

Personnel Services and Multi-Employer Worksite Guidelines

Personnel services firms employ medical care staff and service employees who are assigned to work at hospitals and other healthcare facilities that contract with the firm.

Often the employees are paid by the personnel services firm, but day-to-day supervision of the work is provided by the healthcare facility. When the host employer exercises day-to-day supervision over the personnel service workers, they are the employees of the host employer, as well as of the personnel service.

Under these circumstances the personnel service firm can be held accountable for meeting the following provisions of the standard:

- providing hepatitis B vaccinations;

- managing post-exposure evaluation and follow-up;

- recordkeeping;

- providing generic training;

- exercising reasonable diligence to assure that the host workplace facility is in compliance with the Bloodborne Pathogens Standard; and

- when violations of the standard at the host workplace are known by the firm, the firm takes reasonable steps to have the host employer correct the violation.

The host employer must comply with all provisions of the standard with respect to these workers i.e., providing appropriate engineering controls, an exposure control plan that is explained and available to the worker and personal protective equipment in the appropriate size and type. With regards to Hepatitis B vaccination, post-exposure evaluation and follow-up, recordkeeping, and generic training, the host employer's obligation is to take reasonable measures to assure that the personnel service firm has complied with these provisions.

The shared responsibilities of both employers is referred to as multi-employer worksite guidelines.

Home Health Services

The employees of home health service companies may provide health services in private homes. The employer does not control the private home worksite to which the employee is sent to provide services. Therefore, the application of the bloodborne pathogens standard is restricted in the home health services industry.

This does not mean that the private home worksite is free from bloodborne pathogen hazards. Employees should follow work practice guidelines and use personal protective equipment. Prevention of exposure is the key to protecting your good health.

As a result, OSHA may not cite those employers for site-dependent provisions of the standard when the hazard is site-specific.

OSHA has determined that the employer will not be held responsible for the following site-specific violations (e.g., violations occurring in a private home):

- housekeeping requirements, such as the maintenance of a clean and sanitary worksite;

- the handling and disposal of regulated waste;

- ensuring the use of personal protective equipment;

- ensuring that specific work practices are followed (e.g., handwashing with running water); and

- ensuring the use of engineering controls.

The employer will be held responsible for all non site-specific requirements of the bloodborne pathogens standard, such as:

- the non-site specific requirements of the exposure control plan;

- providing hepatitis B vaccinations;

- post-exposure evaluation, and follow-up;

- recordkeeping;

- providing generic training that is not workplace specific in detail and content; and

- for the provision of appropriate personal protective equipment to employees.

Physicians and Healthcare Professionals in an Independent Practice

In applying the provisions of the bloodborne pathogens standard in situations involving physicians, the status of the physician is important. Physicians may be employers or employees. In this situation, the assignment of responsibilities under the standard is similar to those in effect for personnel services firms.

In general, professional corporations are the employers of their physician-members and must comply with the hepatitis B vaccination, post-exposure evaluation and follow up, recordkeeping and site-specific training provisions, with respect to these physicians when they work at host employer sites. The host employer is not responsible for these provisions with respect to physicians with staff privileges, but the host employer must comply with all other provisions of the standard in accordance with the multi-employer worksite guidelines.

Independent Contractors

Independent contractors are companies that provide a service, such as radiology or housekeeping, to host employers. They provide supervisory and other personnel to carry out the service. Both the companies and the host employers are responsible for complying with all provisions of the standard in accordance with the multi-employer worksite guidelines.

Other Industries

Although these industries are not free from the hazards of bloodborne pathogens, the bloodborne pathogens standard does not apply to the construction, agriculture, marine terminal and longshoring industries.

Good Samaritan Assistance

Employees who do not fall within the scope of this standard may still experience a specific exposure incident at work that is unrelated to the performance of their job duties. An example is "Good Samaritan" assistance, which is voluntarily performed to an injured co-worker or a member of the public.

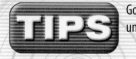

TIPS   Good Samaritan Acts are not covered under the standard.

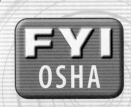

OSHA strongly encourages employers to offer any employee who experiences an exposure incident at work confidential medical evaluation including necessary post exposure prophylaxis and follow-up treatment.

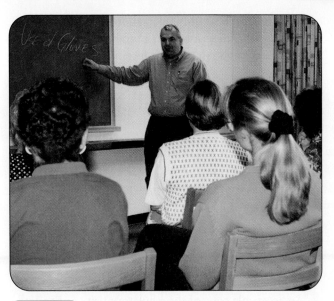

Figure 1-3 Annual training is necessary to ensure employee safety.

Why Do I Need This Manual?

This manual provides OSHA-specific bloodborne pathogens guidelines and is used in conjunction with, and as a supplement to your worksite-specific training. You are encouraged to gather worksite-specific detail on various work pages throughout the manual. Exercises at the end of each chapter help you check what you have learned and how it may be applied to your particular worksite requirements.

This manual will not make you an expert in bloodborne pathogens or the treatment of bloodborne pathogens disease. The detail provided in the manual serves to support the requirements of the OSHA Bloodborne Pathogens Standard. The manual does give you important and necessary information as required by the Standard. Your instructor may expand the information according to worksite specific practices. The categories of information presented in this manual must be included in any and all training.

Meeting OSHA Standards

The goal of training is to educate the employee regarding general bloodborne pathogens issues, as well as how to minimize or eliminate their exposure by a combination of universal precautions, work practice controls, engineering controls and personal protective equipment.

Trainees must have direct access to a qualified trainer during training. Training the employees solely by means of a film, video or computer CD-ROM without the opportunity for a discussion period is not acceptable and constitutes a violation of the Standard. The trainer must be familiar with the manner in which the elements in the training program relate to the workplace practices. This may also be accomplished by having two trainers: one to discuss generic bloodborne pathogens training and one to discuss site-specific information. ▶ **Figure 1-3**

All employees, at the time of initial assignment to tasks with occupational exposure to blood or OPIM, must receive training on the hazards associated with blood and OPIM, and the protective measures to be taken to mini-

mize the risk of occupational exposure prior to actually performing any of the tasks.

Thereafter, training is provided at least annually and must be provided within one year of the original training that occurred prior to the initial work assignment. Whenever a change in an employee's responsibilities, procedures, or work situation is such that an employee's occupational exposure is affected, additional training or, as stated in the CPL, 'retraining' must take place. Retraining is not the same as annual training. Training must occur when new equipment is brought to the worksite that might affect the employee's possible exposure.

Annual training must cover topics listed in the standard to the extent needed and must emphasize new information or procedures. Otherwise, it does need to be an exact repetition of the previous annual training including all the required categories of information and other included site-specific information.

The provisions for employee training are performance oriented, with flexibility in training permitted to allow the program to be tailored to the employee's background and responsibilities or other site-specific needs. The categories of information presented in this manual must be included in any and all training.

OSHA requires that any training (including written material, oral presentations, films, video tapes, computer programs or audio tapes) be presented in a manner appropriate to the employee's education, literacy level, and language. If an employee is only proficient in a language other than English, the trainer or an interpreter must convey the information in that language.

It is necessary to record information about the dates of training sessions, a summary of the training content and the names and job titles of the employees who attend the training.

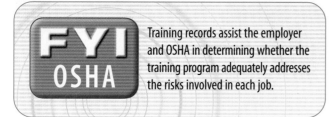

Training records assist the employer and OSHA in determining whether the training program adequately addresses the risks involved in each job.

OSHA Required Categories of Information

A. An accessible copy of the regulatory text (Appendix A) and an explanation of its contents (this manual)

B. A general explanation of the epidemiology and symptoms of bloodborne disease (Chapter 2)

C. An explanation of the modes of transmission of bloodborne pathogens (Chapter 2)

D. An explanation of the employer's Exposure Control Plan and the means by which the employee can obtain a copy of the written plan (supplied by your company directly or through the instructor) (Chapter 4)

E. An explanation of the appropriate methods for recognizing tasks and other activities that may involve exposure to blood and other potentially infectious materials (Chapter 3)

F. An explanation of the use and limitations of methods that will prevent or reduce exposure including appropriate engineering controls, work practices, and personal protective equipment (Chapter 3)

G. Information on the types, proper use, location, removal, handling, decontamination, and disposal of personal protective equipment (Chapter 3)

H. An explanation of the basis for selection of personal protective equipment (Chapter 3)

I. Information on the Hepatitis B vaccine, including information on its efficacy, safety, method of administration, the benefits of being vaccinated, and that the vaccine and vaccination will be offered free of charge to employees covered by the standard (Chapter 2)

J. Information on the appropriate actions to take and persons to contact in an emergency (*exposure outside the normal scope of work*) involving blood or other potentially infectious materials (Chapter 2)

K. An explanation of the procedure to follow if an exposure incident occurs including the method of reporting the incident and the medical follow-up that will be made available (Chapter 2)

L. Information on the post-exposure evaluation and follow-up that the employer is required to provide for the employee following an exposure incident (Chapter 2)

M. An explanation of the signs, labels, and/or color-coding required (Chapter 3)

N. An opportunity for interactive questions and answers with the person conducting the training session (during and after training session)

The Ryan White Act

The CDC is in the process of preparing the final list of diseases required by the passage of the Public Law 101-381, the Ryan White Comprehensive AIDS Resources Emergency Act. The Act creates a notification system for emergency response employees listed as police, fire, and EMS, who are exposed to diseases such as *M. tuberculosis,* Hepatitis B or C, and HIV.

Site-Specific Work Page

EMPLOYEE TRAINING

Date/Time of Training _____

Training Location _____

Your Name _____

This bloodborne pathogens training has been conducted by: _____

Attach a few comments about his or her qualifications.

_____

_____

Name of your supervisor or other responsible person you would contact in the event of an exposure.

_____

BBP Training materials are available at _____

This is: Initial training: ❑ Yes   ❑ No

           Retraining: ❑ Yes   ❑ No

           Annual training: ❑ Yes   ❑ No

This training occurred during my routine work hours: ❑ Yes   ❑ No

This training occurred at no cost to me: ❑ Yes   ❑ No

A copy of the Standard is included in my Bloodborne Pathogens manual: ❑ Yes   ❑ No

The training materials used by the instructor are easy for me to understand: ❑ Yes   ❑ No

The training materials used are in a language I understand: ❑ Yes   ❑ No

Terms are defined in Appendix A of my Bloodborne Pathogens manual: ❑ Yes   ❑ No

My company's Exposure Control Plan is available at: _____

Training records are available for 3 years and are kept by: _____

I may request a copy of my training record from: _____

Request for a copy of my training record is to be provided within 15 days: ❑ Yes   ❑ No

Training records are not considered confidential: ❑ Yes   ❑ No

Questions about the Standard were answered by the trainer: ❑ Yes   ❑ No

My question about the OSHA Bloodborne Pathogens Standard is:

_____

_____

Learning Activities

1. What kind of task would require training in bloodborne pathogens and OPIM safety?

   _____

   _____

   _____

   _____

   _____

   _____

   _____

   _____

T   F   2. An explanation of the symptoms caused by bloodborne pathogens is not a site-specific topic.

T   F   3. Information about the locations of the eye wash stations is a site-specific topic.

T   F   4. Recommending and participating in the selection of engineering controls or personal protective equipment is an example of site-specific information.

Yes   No   5. Is there any industry free from the hazards of bloodborne pathogens?

                6. Name an industry not covered by the OSHA Bloodborne Pathogens Standard.

   _____

   _____

Yes   No   7. If there is a change to my work practices that would change my exposure to bloodborne pathogens, I would receive retraining.

Yes   No   8. I must receive training every year.

Yes   No   9. OSHA requires the use of engineering controls.

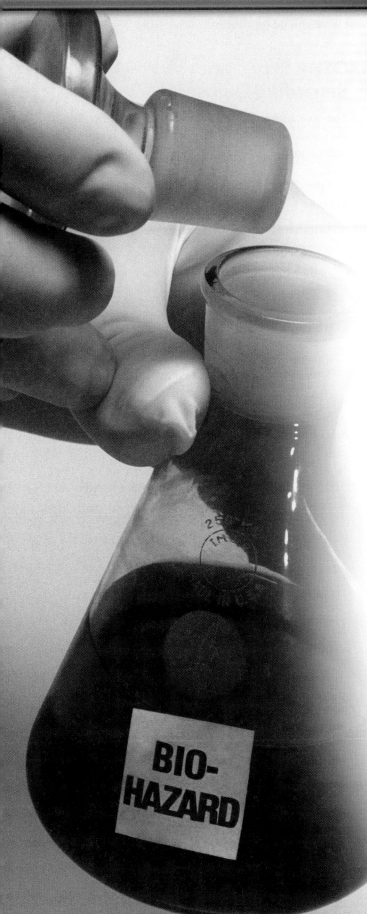

Chapter 2

Bloodborne Pathogens

Overview

Occupational exposure to blood or OPIM means that you are at risk for infection from disease causing organisms that may be transmitted through direct contact with blood or OPIM. The hazard of exposure to infected blood or OPIM is not restricted to the healthcare industry.

The likelihood of becoming infected after a single exposure to blood containing a disease-causing organism depends upon many factors. The factors most commonly associated with transmission of disease include the presence of the organism in the source blood or OPIM; the type of injury or contact sustained by you (e.g., splash or puncture wound); the viral level present in the source individual and, your current health (e.g., immunized against Hepatitis B).

There are many bloodborne pathogens. The likelihood of being exposed to a particular disease-causing organism varies and is affected by:

1. The geographic region where the work occurs (i.e., certain countries and/or areas have a much higher incidence of diseases caused by bloodborne pathogens). It is estimated that 16-18 million people in Central and South America are infected with Typanosoma curzi. This is a bloodborne pathogen parasite responsible for Chagas disease.

2. The type of work performed (e.g., work in a research lab that investigates and cultures various viruses and bacteria may increase the risk).

It is not possible to include every possible bloodborne pathogen in this manual, therefore, the emphasis in this section is on HBV, HCV and HIV. The Standard includes **any** pathogenic microorganism that may be present in human blood or OPIM and can infect and cause disease in persons who are exposed to blood containing the pathogen.

Your employer should determine the inclusion of information about other bloodborne pathogens in your training based on your geographic location and type of potential exposure. For example, if you work in facilities that are located near or along the border with Mexico and you might reasonably expect to have occupational exposure to the blood of people from Mexico or Central America, then it might be important to learn more about Chagas disease.

What Are Bloodborne Pathogens?

Bloodborne pathogens are disease-causing microorganisms (e.g., viruses, bacteria, and parasites) that may be present in human blood. They may be transmitted with any exposure to blood or OPIM.

Mode of Transmission of Bloodborne Pathogens

Bloodborne pathogens are transmitted when blood or OPIM come in contact with mucous membranes or non-intact skin. Non-intact skin includes, but is not limited to, cuts, abrasions, burns, rashes, acne, paper cuts, and hangnails. Bloodborne pathogens may also be transmitted by blood splash or spray, handling or touching contaminated items or surfaces and injection under the skin by puncture wounds or cuts from contaminated sharps.

▼ Figure 2-1

The majority of occupational HIV transmission has occurred through puncture injury. However, there have been documented HIV transmissions from non-sexual, non-percutaneous exposures to fresh blood or body fluid contaminated with HIV. Transmission has been documented to occur after contact with HIV-contaminated blood through non-intact skin and mucous membranes.

One worker became HIV positive after a splash of HIV contaminated blood to the eyes. Contact with blood or OPIM should be avoided.

OSHA Expectations Regarding Exposure

The objective of the Standard is to minimize or eliminate the hazard posed by exposure to blood or OPIM. However, occupational exposure to a bloodborne pathogen may occur.

If there is a risk of exposure or injury, it is important to know:

1. if there is a way to prevent infection as a result of exposure to the pathogen (e.g., immunization),

2. the symptoms caused by infection with the pathogen, as well as the natural course of the infection,

3. that counseling specific to the exposure incident is available and,

4. the post-exposure treatments and follow-up that may be provided.

If you are exposed to bloodborne pathogens, a confidential medical evaluation is to be made **immediately** available to you, the injured employee. The word "immediately" is used in the Standard to emphasize the importance of prompt medical evaluation and prophylaxis. An exact time cannot be stated because the time limit on the effectiveness of post-exposure prophylactic measures does vary depending on the infection of concern.

Medical evaluation must be confidential, protect your identity and test results.

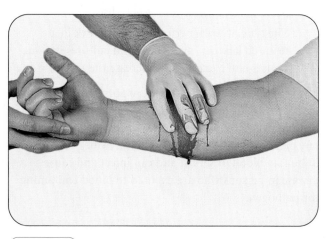

Figure 2-1) Always wear gloves to prevent contamination.

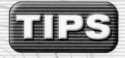

- Needle stick and other sharps injuries are primarily associated with the following activities: disposing needles; administering injections; drawing blood, including use of glass capillary tubes; recapping needles; and handling trash and dirty linens.

- The employer does not have a specific right to know the actual results of the source individual's blood testing, but must ensure that the information is provided to the evaluating healthcare professional.

If you go for a medical evaluation the following information will be made available to the health professional.

1. A copy of the OSHA guidelines section 1910.1030

2. A description of how the incident occurred as it relates to your employment

3. The results of the source individual's testing (if available)

4. All medical records that are relevant for your proper treatment (if treatment is necessary), including a copy of your Hepatitis B vaccination status with the dates of all the Hepatitis B vaccinations and any medical records relative to the your ability to receive the vaccination

You and your employer should expect that current CDC guidelines will be used to guide post-exposure prophylaxis and treatment.

It is the employer's responsibility to ensure that your medical records are kept confidential. Your records cannot be disclosed without your express written consent to any person within or outside the workplace except as required by law. Your employer will have a copy of the healthcare provider's written opinion regarding the incident.

During consultation with the health professional, decisions will be made about the need for Hepatitis B vaccination, laboratory tests, and information will be provided about available post-exposure prophylaxis and treatments.

The healthcare professional will discuss the laboratory test results with you. A plan will be created that identifies any necessary follow-up or treatments including initiation of Hepatitis B immunization, if Hepatitis B vaccine is indicated. Any post-exposure treatments and follow-up plans should be in accordance with the current CDC guidelines.

TIPS

- Confidentiality requirements must be part of any contract with a health professional, health clinic, or other healthcare facility that provides post exposure evaluation or follow-up treatment programs.

- It is possible to test the blood for antibodies specific to HBV, HBC, and HIV.

- Test interpretation occurs in consultation with your healthcare professional and is beyond the scope of this training.

Reporting Requirements

Emergency Measures in the Event of an Exposure

- If you have an exposure incident to another person's blood or OPIM, immediately wash the exposed area with warm water and soap.

- If the exposed area was in your mouth, rinse your mouth with water or mouthwash (whichever is most readily available).

- If the exposure was in your eyes, flush with warm water (or normal saline if available). A quick rinse is probably not adequate, you want to irrigate the area completely with water.

- Your employer will have site-specific work practices to follow in event of an emergency.

What Is an Occupational Exposure Incident?

An occupational exposure incident occurs if you are in a work situation and come in contact with blood or OPIM.

For OSHA 2000 record-keeping purposes, an occupational bloodborne pathogens exposure incident (e.g., needlestick, laceration, or splash) shall be classified as an injury since it is usually the result of an instantaneous event or exposure. ▼ Figure 2-2

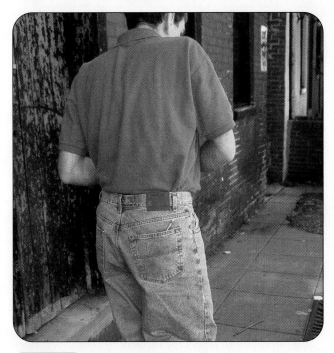

Figure 2-2 An uncapped needle can cause an injury.

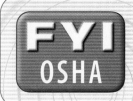

OSHA requires that information on the appropriate actions to take and persons to contact in an emergency involving blood or OPIM be provided as part of BBP training.

Once an occupational exposure to blood or other potentially infectious materials has occurred, the employee's name and job classification are listed on the OSHA 200 log. A review of the job classification should be undertaken and determination made as to which emploees, if any, in that classification should now be covered under the Standard.

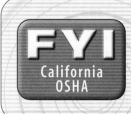

Califorina OSHA requires a sharps injury log, which records the date and time of each sharps injury resulting in an exposure incident, as well as, the type and brand of device involved in the exposure incident.

Assessing Exposure Determination

The employer must identify and document the job classifications in which all employees have occupational exposure and/or where some employees have an occupational exposure. The exposure determination must have been made without taking into consideration the use of personal protective clothing or equipment. The Exposure Control Plan should identify the person responsible for the determination and assessment of an exposure incident.

Reporting an Incident

The goal of reporting an incident is to assure timely access to medical services and to identify and adopt other methods or devices to prevent exposure incidents from recurring.

At sites where an exposure incident has occurred it should be determined if the procedures were properly followed through interviews, incident report reviews, and, if necessary, medical records reviews.

The documentation of circumstances surrounding an incident allows identification and correction of hazards. To be useful, the documentation should contain sufficient detail about the incident.

It is important to report the incident to your supervisor. OSHA requires you to report the following information:

- date and time of the exposure incident
- job classification of the exposed employee
- work site location where the exposure incident occurred;
- work practices being followed
- engineering controls in use at the time including a description of the device in use (e.g., type and brand of sharp involved in the exposure incident)
- protective equipment or clothing that was used at the time of the exposure incident
- procedure being performed when the incident occurred
- your training for the activity.

California OSHA also requires:

- identifying the body part involved in the exposure incident.
- the engineering controls in use at the time if the sharp had engineered sharps injury protection
- whether the protective mechanism was activated, and whether the injury occurred before the protective mechanism was activated, during activation of the mechanism or after activation of the mechanism, if applicable
- if the sharp had no engineered sharps injury protection, the injured employee's opinion as to whether and how such a mechanism could have prevented the injury
- the employee's opinion about whether any other engineering, administrative or work practice control could have prevented the injury

Once an incident has been reported, your employer will take the following steps:

1. identify and document the source individual, and
2. obtain consent and make arrangements to have the source individual tested as soon as possible to determine HIV, HCV, and HBV infectivity.

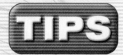

- It may not be feasible to identify the source individual.
- State laws may vary; please check with your instructor regarding testing and test result confidentiality laws in your state.

Examples of when you may be unable to identify the source individual include needlesticks caused by unmarked syringes left in laundry, or those involving blood samples which are not properly labeled, as well as incidents occurring where state or local laws prohibit such identification.

As stated before, the source individual's blood (if available) may be tested for HBV, HCV, and/or HIV and the results of the test will be made known to you. Testing of the source individual's blood may be performed after consent is obtained. It should be documented when legally required consent to test the blood is not obtained.

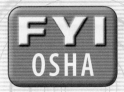
OSHA does not require redrawing of the source individual's blood specifically for HBV, HCV and HIV testing without the consent of the source individual.

Your blood may be tested for HBV, HCV and/or HIV only with your consent. You may refuse. Counseling and evaluation of reported illnesses are not dependent on you choosing to have baseline HBV, HCV and HIV serological testing.

You may choose to have your blood drawn and stored for 90 days. If you change your mind within the 90 days, testing will be done. The 90-day time frame allows you the opportunity to obtain knowledge about baseline serologic testing after exposure incidents, and to participate in further discussion, education or counseling. If you elect not to have the blood tested, the sample will be disposed of without testing after 90 days.

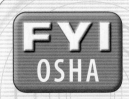
OSHA encourages employees to consent to blood collection at the time of exposure.

Specific Bloodborne Pathogens
Hepatitis Viruses

Hepatitis means "inflammation of the liver." A number of things including drugs, poisons and other toxins, and bloodborne pathogens may cause hepatitis. This section will focus on two causes of viral hepatitis that are important in the United States – Hepatitis B Virus (HBV) and Hepatitis C Virus (HCV).

FIRST AID PROVIDERS

The employer's exposure control plan must specifically address the provisions of the Standard as they apply to **first aid providers.**

The Exposure Control Plan must include:

- Provision for a reporting procedure that ensures that all first aid incidents involving the presence of blood or OPIM will be reported to the employer before the end of the work shift during which the incident occurred.

- The report must include the names of all first aid providers who rendered assistance, regardless of whether personal protective equipment was used and must describe the first aid incident, including time and date. The description must include a determination of whether or not, in addition to the presence of blood or other potentially infectious materials, an "exposure incident," as defined by the standard, occurred. This determination is necessary in order to ensure that the proper post-exposure evaluation, prophylaxis, and follow-up procedures required by the standard are made available immediately, whenever there has been an "exposure incident" as defined by the standard.

- A report that lists all such first aid incidents, that is readily available, upon request, to all employees and to the Assistant Secretary.

- Provision for the bloodborne pathogens training program for designated first aid providers to include the specifics of this reporting procedure.

- Provision for the full hepatitis B vaccination series to be made available as soon as possible, but in no event later than 24 hours, to all unvaccinated first aid providers who have rendered assistance in any situation involving the presence of blood or OPIM, regardless of whether or not a specific "exposure incident," as defined by the standard, has occurred.

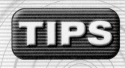
Infection with one form of hepatitis does not prevent infection with another form of hepatitis. For example, a person with an HCV infection may still get an HBV infection.

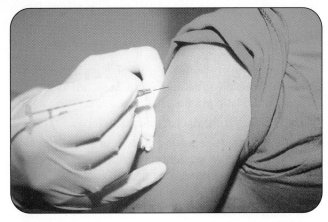

Figure 2-3   Immunization against HBV is possible.

Hepatitis B Virus

Hepatitis B virus can affect anyone. Each year, in the United States, 140,000-320,000 people will become infected with the virus. Studies conducted by the CDC have shown a steady decline in the incidence of HBV. This decline is attributed to the widespread use of Hepatitis B vaccine and the implementation of other prevention methods such as engineering and work practice controls, personal protective equipment, and universal precautions.

Even though there has been a decline in the number of infections with HBV, the CDC estimated that in 1994, 1024 health care workers became infected with the virus. Sadly, it is projected that of this group, 22 persons will suffer significant disease and eventually die from complications related to the infection. It is estimated that 1-1.25 million Americans are chronically infected with HBV.

Prevention and Control

The hepatitis B vaccine has been available since 1982. The vaccine does not contain any live components. The vaccine is given in a series of 3 shots.

HBV Immunization

All people who have routine occupational exposure to blood or other potentially infectious materials have the right to receive the immunization series against Hepatitis B at no personal expense. The standard includes temporary, part-time workers and volunteers. (▲ Figure 2-3)

There are several reasons why you may choose not to receive the Hepatitis B vaccine. Among the most common reasons are:

1. documentation exists that you have previously received the series,

2. antibody testing reveals that you are immune,

3. medical evaluation shows that vaccination is contraindicated, or

4. you are allergic to any component of the vaccine.

Exception for Hepatitis B Vaccination

Designated first aid providers who have occupational exposure are not required to be offered pre-exposure hepatitis B vaccine if the following conditions exist:

1. The primary job assignment of the designated first aid provider is not the rendering of first aid.

2. Any first aid rendered by the first aid provider is rendered only as a collateral duty responding solely to injuries resulting from workplace incidents, and generally at the location where the incident occurred.

3. This provision does not apply to designated first aid providers who render assistance on a regular basis, for example, at a first aid station, clinic, dispensary, or other location where injured employees routinely go for such assistance, and emergency or public safety personnel who are expected to render first aid in the course of their work.

Prescreening, antibody testing, is not required, and your employer may not make prescreening a requirement for receiving the vaccine. If an employer wishes prescreening, it must be made available to you at no cost. If you choose to have prescreening, the testing must be done at an accredited laboratory.

The standard requires that your employer offer the vaccine at a convenient time and place to you, during normal work hours. If travel is required away from the worksite, your employer is responsible for that cost. The standard includes temporary and part-time workers.

Your employer cannot require you to pay for testing and then reimburse you if you remain employed for a specific time. Nor are you required to reimburse your employer for the cost of the vaccine if you leave your job.

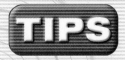

TIPS

- Immunization with Hepatitis B vaccine should be made available within 10 working days of initial assignment to the job.

- Your employer cannot require you to use your health insurance or your family insurance to pay for the cost of the vaccine.

- To learn more about CDC recommendations visit: http://www.cdc.gov

While it is OSHA's intent to have the employer remove, as much as possible, obstacles to your acceptance of the vaccine, the term "made available" emphasizes that you may refuse the series by signing the Hepatitis B vaccine declination form (Appendix C). If you change your mind while still covered under the standard at a later date, you may still receive the vaccine at no cost.

If your job requires you to have ongoing contact with patients or blood and you are at ongoing risk for injuries with sharp instruments or needlesticks, the CDC recommends that you be tested for antibody to Hepatitis B surface antigen (HBsAg), one to two months after the completion of the three-dose vaccination series. If you do not respond to the primary vaccination series you must be re-vaccinated with a second three-dose vaccine series and re-tested for HBsAg. Non-responders must be medically evaluated.

Contraindications

- You should not receive the vaccine if you are sensitive to yeast or any other component of the vaccine.

- Consultation with a physician is required for persons with heart disease, fever, or other illness.

- If you are pregnant or breastfeeding an infant, you should consult your physician before receiving the vaccine.

Side Effects of the Vaccine

The side effects of the vaccine are minimal and may include localized swelling, pain, bruising, or redness at the injection site. The most common systemic reactions include flu-like symptoms such as fatigue, weakness, headache, fever, or malaise.

About the Vaccines

Recombivax HB provided by Merck Sharp & Dohme or Engerix-B by Smith-Kline, Inc. are the vaccines used to prevent infection with the hepatitis B virus. The vaccine against hepatitis B, prepared from recombinant yeast cultures, is free of association with human blood or blood products. A new (1999) single-antigen hepatitis B vaccine does not contain thimerosal as a preservative.

The vaccine is given in three doses over a six-month period; the first is given at an agreed-on date, the second is given one month later, and the third dose is given five months after the second dose. The vaccine is administered by needle into a large muscle such as the deltoid in the upper arm. However, for persons at risk of hemorrhage following intramuscular injection, the vaccine may be administered subcutaneously.

In persons receiving the vaccine, 87 percent will develop immunity after the second dose of the vaccine, and 96 percent will develop immunity after the third dose.

Clinical Features and History of Hepatitis B

The symptoms of HBV infection typically last four to six weeks and include:

- Jaundice (your eyes or skin may turn yellow)
- fatigue
- abdominal pain
- loss of appetite
- intermittent nausea
- vomiting

It is expected that 70,000 to 160,000 people will develop symptomatic infections with HBV and 8,400 to 19,000 of these people will require hospitalization. Unfortunately, each year, as many as 320 will die from the acute infection with HBV.

The incubation period for HBV (the time from exposure to developing the disease) averages twelve weeks, with a range of four weeks to six months. In the majority, 90-94% of the cases, infection with HBV resolves without further complication. However, about 8,000-32,000 (6%-10%) of all the annual infections will progress and suffer chronic infection with HBV. Over time, chronic infection causes significant injury to the liver. 5,000 - 6,000 deaths occur each year from chronic HBV liver disease.

Post-Exposure Prophylaxis and Follow-Up for Hepatitis B

There is no cure for infection with HBV. Hepatitis B vaccination is the best protection.

All decisions about post-exposure prophylaxis are made in consultation with your health care professional.

Post-exposure treatment for HBV infection should begin within 24 hours and no later than 7 days.

The post-exposure treatments available include:

1. Hepatitis B immunization, and

2. the use of immune globulin, which has been shown to be effective for passive immunization against HBV if given within hours after the exposure incident.

The decision to provide post-exposure prophylaxis takes into account:

1. whether the source of the blood is available

2. the HbsAg status of the source blood and

3. the hepatitis B vaccination and vaccine-response status of the exposed employee

For any occupational exposure to blood or OPIM of a person not previously vaccinated, hepatitis B vaccination is recommended.

The CDC reports that for an unvaccinated person, the risk from a single needlestick or cut exposure to HBV infected blood ranges from 6-30% and depends on the hepatitis B e antigen (HBeAg) status of the source blood.

Chronic HBV infection treatment options include anti-viral medications and/or liver transplantation.

Hepatitis C Virus

Hepatitis C virus (HCV) infection is the most common chronic bloodborne infection in the United States. HCV is transmitted primarily through large or repeated direct percutaneous exposures to blood.

The incidence of HCV infection has declined. Transfusion-associated cases occurred prior to donor screening and are now very rare. Injecting-drug use consistently has accounted for a substantial proportion of HCV infections and currently accounts for 60% of HCV transmission in the United States.

It is estimated that 3.9 million (1.8%) Americans have been infected with HCV of whom 2.7 million are chronically infected. 36,000 new infections occur in the United States each year.

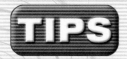

- Hepatitis C (HCV) has specifically been identified wherever HIV and HBV are mentioned in the regulation.

- The CDC reports that the prevalence of HCV infection among health-care workers is no greater than the general population, averaging 1%–2%, and is 10 times lower than the prevalence of HBV infection among health-care workers.

- Needle-stick injury is the only occupational risk factor that has been associated with HCV infection.

- Referral to a specialist in liver disease may be necessary to properly manage an infection with HCV.

- In follow-up studies of health-care workers who sustained percutaneous exposures to blood from anti-HCV positive patients, the incidence of anti-HCV conversion averaged 3.5%.

Prevention and Control

There is no vaccination for HCV.

Prevention recommendations are directed toward the use of engineering and work practice controls, personal protective equipment, and universal precautions.

Clinical Features and History of Hepatitis C

Most patients (70-75%) with acute hepatitis C are asymptomatic. Symptoms may include:

- Jaundice (your eyes or skin may turn yellow)

- fatigue

- abdominal pain

- loss of appetite

- intermittent nausea

- vomiting

The incubation period (the time from exposure to developing the disease) averages seven weeks (range, 3-20 weeks). Chronic infection is common, affecting more than 85% of people infected. Chronic liver disease may occur in 70% of those infected with HCV. It is estimated that 8,000 to 10,000 deaths occur each year as a result of HCV-associated liver disease. HCV is the major cause of liver disease requiring liver transplantation.

Post-Exposure Prophylaxis and Follow-Up

There is no cure for infection with HVC.

All decisions about post-exposure laboratory testing and prophylaxis are made in consultation with your health care professional. The test for HCV and liver function tests should occur as soon as possible after exposure and repeated at four and six months after the exposure.

Currently there is no recommendation for post-exposure prophylaxis of HCV. Immune globulin **is not** effective in providing passive immunization against the disease.

When HCV infection is identified early, referral for medical management to a specialist knowledgeable in this disease is recommended. Limited data indicates that antiviral therapy might be beneficial when started early in the course of the HCV infection. However, no guidelines currently exist for the use of antiviral medications in the acute phase of the infection.

The CDC reports that the risk for infection after a needlestick or cut exposure to HCV-infected blood is about 1.8%.

Chronic HCV infection treatment options include anti-viral medications and liver transplantation.

Human Immunodeficiency Virus

Two types of the human immunodeficiency virus are identified (HIV-1 and HIV-2). Both HIV-1 and HIV-2 are the cause of AIDS; have the same mode of transmission; and are associated with opportunistic infections.

The differences between HIV-1 and HIV-2 should be noted. HIV-2 AIDS develops more slowly and may be milder. There are few reported cases of HIV-2 in the United States. HIV-2 is predominately found in Africa. Hereafter, all references to HIV mean HIV-1.

The CDC reports that in the United States there are 113,167 persons living with HIV infection and there are 299,944 persons living with AIDS. The annual rate of infection with HIV is 16.5 cases per 100,000 population.

▼ Figure 2-4

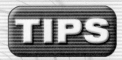

- The CDC is aware of 56 healthcare workers in the United States who have documented HIV seroconversion following occupational exposure. Of the 56 workers, 48 were exposed through percutaneous injuries.

- Of the adults reported with AIDS in the United States through December 1999, 22,218 had been employed in healthcare.

- The CDC is also aware of 136 other cases of HIV infection or AIDS among healthcare workers who have not reported other risk factors for HIV infection and who have reported a history of occupational exposure to blood, body fluids or HIV-infected laboratory material.

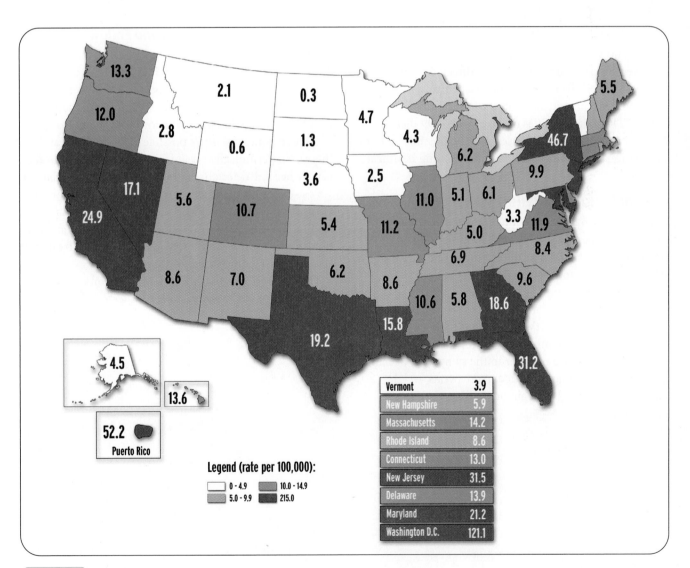

Figure 2-4 AIDS Prevalence Map

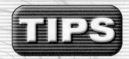

Risk of HIV Infection from Percutaneous Exposure

The average risk for HIV infection from all types of reported percutaneous exposure to HIV infected blood is 0.3%.

The risk is increased in exposures involving:

- deep injury to healthcare worker
- visible blood on the device causing the injury
- a device previously placed in the source patients vein or artery
- a source patient who died as a result of AIDS within 60 days post-exposure

TIPS

- Advances in the field of antiviral therapy and the use of protease inhibitors might change the recommendations for treatment and follow-up for HCV and HIV infection, therefore, it is important to work closely with your healthcare professional and use current CDC guidelines.
- All the antiviral drugs have been associated with significant side effects. Protease inhibitors may interact with other medications and cause serious side effects.

Prevention and Control

There is no vaccination for HIV.

Prevention recommendations are directed toward the use of engineering and work practice controls, personal protective equipment, and universal precautions.

The CDC reports that as of December 1999 there have been 56 documented cases and 136 possible cases of occupationally acquired HIV infection among healthcare workers.

Clinical Features and History of HIV

The only way to determine for sure whether you are infected is to be tested. The incubation period with HIV from the time of HIV infection to the development of AIDS may take 8 to 10 years. This time varies greatly from person to person.

You cannot rely on symptoms to know whether or not you are infected with HIV. Many people who are infected with HIV experience no symptoms for many years. The symptoms of AIDS are similar to the symptoms of many of infections and might include night sweats, weight loss, fever, fatigue, gland pain or swelling, and muscle or joint pain.

Post Exposure Prophylaxis and Follow-Up for HIV

There is no cure for infection with HIV.

All decisions about post-exposure laboratory testing and prophylaxis are made in consultation with your healthcare professional. Testing for the HIV antibody should be done as soon as possible after exposure and, thereafter, periodically for at least six months. Antibodies usually become detectable within three months of infection.

Post-exposure treatment is **not** recommended for all occupational exposures. 99.7% of the exposures do not lead to HIV infection. If treatment with antiviral medications plus a protease inhibitor is recommended, treatment should begin within hours of the exposure.

The CDC reports that the risk of infection after a needlestick or cut exposure to HIV-infected blood is about 0.3%.

Site-Specific Work Page

In addition to HBV, HBC, and HIV, the instructor also reviewed the following bloodborne pathogens.

Pathogen: _____

Prevention and Control: _____

Clinical Features and History of the Disease: _____

Post-Exposure Prophylaxis and Follow-up: _____

Pathogen: _____

Prevention and Control: _____

Clinical Features and History of the Disease: _____

Post-Exposure Prophylaxis and Follow-up: _____

Pathogen: _____

Prevention and Control: _____

Clinical Features and History of the Disease: _____

Post-Exposure Prophylaxis and Follow-up: _____

The required medical records are maintained by: _____

at (location) _____

Medical records are kept for the duration of my employment plus 30 years: ❑ Yes   ❑ No

Medical care at my worksite is provided by: _____

Medical records are provided to you or to anyone having written consent from you within 15 days: ❑ True   ❑ False

The person responsible to evaluate if an exposure incident meets OSHA record keeping requirements is:

_____

Hepatitis B vaccine is provided by _____ at (location) _____ .

The health professional's written opinion concerning Hepatitis B immunization is limited to whether the employee requires the vaccine and whether the vaccine was administered.   ❑ True   ❑ False

My question about Hepatitis B is: _____

My question about Hepatitis C is: _____

My question about HIV is: _____

My question about another bloodborne pathogen is: _____

Learning Activities

_____ C _____ **1.** For which virus is there an effective vaccine.
   a. HIV
   b. HCV
   c. HBV

(T) F **2.** If you do not respond to the first HBV immunization series you may be re-vaccinnated with a second series.

3. List two symptoms of hepatitis.

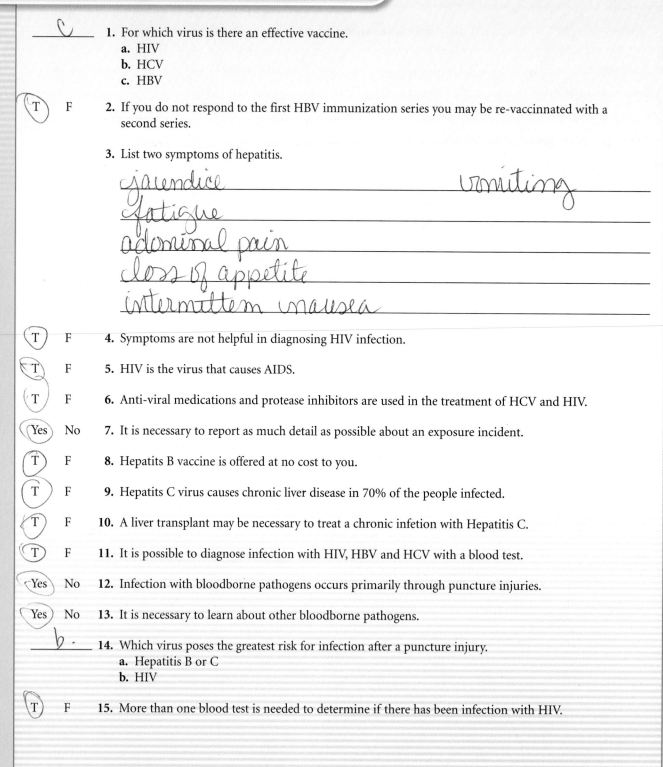

jaundice   vomiting
fatigue
abdominal pain
loss of appetite
intermittem nausea

(T) F **4.** Symptoms are not helpful in diagnosing HIV infection.

(T) F **5.** HIV is the virus that causes AIDS.

(T) F **6.** Anti-viral medications and protease inhibitors are used in the treatment of HCV and HIV.

(Yes) No **7.** It is necessary to report as much detail as possible about an exposure incident.

(T) F **8.** Hepatits B vaccine is offered at no cost to you.

(T) F **9.** Hepatits C virus causes chronic liver disease in 70% of the people infected.

(T) F **10.** A liver transplant may be necessary to treat a chronic infetion with Hepatitis C.

(T) F **11.** It is possible to diagnose infection with HIV, HBV and HCV with a blood test.

(Yes) No **12.** Infection with bloodborne pathogens occurs primarily through puncture injuries.

(Yes) No **13.** It is necessary to learn about other bloodborne pathogens.

_____ b. _____ **14.** Which virus poses the greatest risk for infection after a puncture injury.
   a. Hepatitis B or C
   b. HIV

(T) F **15.** More than one blood test is needed to determine if there has been infection with HIV.

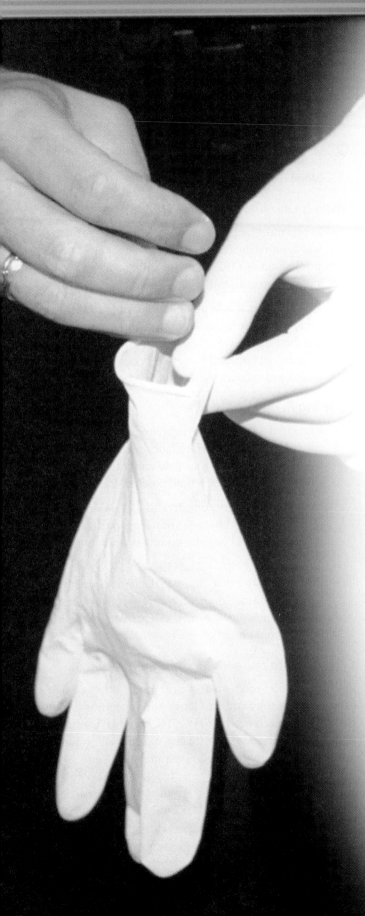

Chapter 3

Prevention

Overview

OSHA defines four principal strategies to prevent or reduce exposure to bloodborne pathogens. These strategies are used in combination to offer you maximum protection. It is OSHA's view that preventing exposures requires a comprehensive program, including engineering controls (e.g., needleless devices, shielded needle devices, and plastic capillary tubes) and proper work practices (e.g., no-hands procedures in handling contaminated sharps). If engineering and work practice controls do not eliminate exposure, the use of personal protective equipment (e.g., eye protection) and universal precautions are required.

Your employer's Exposure Control Plan describes the engineering controls in use at your worksite. Significant improvements in technology are most evident in the growing market of safer medical devices that minimize, control, or prevent exposure incidents. Employee participation in the selection of new devices is encouraged but not required by OSHA. OSHA does not advocate the use of one particular device over another. An annual review of your employer's Exposure Plan should include identification of new safety devices. Adoption of engineering controls requires changes to your employer's Exposure Control Plan and retraining in the proper use of the control.

According to California OSHA, the use of needleless systems, needle devices with engineered sharps injury protection, and non-needle sharps with engineered sharps injury protection is required except under four conditions:

1. lack of market availability

2. information that the device will jeopardize patient care

3. information indicating that the device is not more effective in reducing sharps injuries than the device currently used by the employer

4. lack of sufficient information to determine whether a new device on the market will effectively reduce the chances of a sharps injury

When occupational exposure remains after using engineering and work practice controls, employers must provide personal protective equipment. Personal protective equipment is used to protect you from contamination of skin, mucous membranes, or puncture wounds. Universal Precautions is a strategy to structure your approach to working with all human blood and certain body fluids. All these strategies combined promote worker safety and provide a safer working environment.

Engineering Controls

Engineering controls attempt to design safety into the tools and workspace organization. Examples include handwashing facilities, eye stations, sharps containers, biohazard labels, self-sheathing needles on syringes and needleless IV systems.

TIPS Where engineering controls will reduce employee exposure either by removing, eliminating or isolating the hazard, they must be used.

Your employer is responsible for the full cost of instituting engineering and work practice controls. Your employer is also responsible to regularly examine and repair and/or replace engineering controls as often as necessary to ensure that each control is maintained and that it provides the protection intended. Regularly scheduled inspections are required to confirm, for instance, that engineering controls such as safer devices continue to function effectively, that protective shields have not been removed or broken, and that physical, mechanical or replacement-dependent controls are functioning as intended. Your employer may assign this task to you.

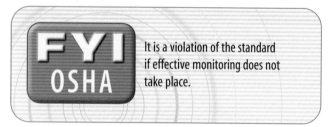

FYI OSHA It is a violation of the standard if effective monitoring does not take place.

Work practice controls shall be evaluated and updated on a regular schedule to ensure their effectiveness.

Labeling Regulated Waste

What is Regulated Waste?

The term "regulated waste" refers to the following categories of waste which require special handling, at a minimum:

- liquid or semi-liquid blood or OPIM

- items contaminated with blood or OPIM and which would release these substances in a liquid or semi-liquid state if compressed

- items that are caked with dried blood or OPIM and are capable of releasing these materials during handling

- contaminated sharps

- pathological and microbiological wastes containing blood or OPIM

When Is Labeling Regulated Waste Necessary?

- Labels must be provided on containers of regulated waste, on refrigerators and freezers that are used to store blood or OPIM, and on containers used to store, dispose of, transport, or ship blood or OPIM.

- Equipment that is being sent to another facility for servicing or decontamination must have a label attached stating which portions of the equipment remain contaminated to warn other employees of the hazard and encourage them to use proper precautions.

Labeling Regulated Waste

- Regulated waste containers are required to be labeled with the biohazard label or color-coded to warn employees who may have contact with the containers of the potential hazard posed by their contents.

- Even if your facility considers all of its waste to be regulated waste, the waste containers must still bear the required label or color-coding in order to protect new employees and employees from outside facilities.

- Regulated waste that has been decontaminated need not be labeled or color-coded. However, your employer must have controls in place to determine if the decontamination process is successful.

Exceptions to Labeling Requirements

Blood and blood products that bear an identifying label as specified by the Food and Drug Administration and that have been screened for HBV, HCV and HIV antibodies and released for transfusion or other clinical uses are exempted from the labeling requirements.

When blood is being drawn or laboratory procedures are being performed on blood samples, then the individual containers housing the blood or OPIM do not have to be labeled provided the larger container into which they are placed for storage, transport, shipment, or disposal (for example, a test tube rack) is labeled.

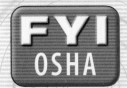

When there is an overlap between the OSHA mandated label and the DOT required label, the DOT label will be considered acceptable on the outside of the transport container, provided that the OSHA mandated label appears on any internal containers which may be present.

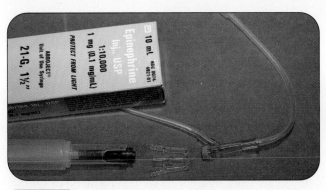

Figure 3-2 Needleless system

Biohazard Labels

Biohazard labels may be attached to bags containing potentially infectious materials. These labels must be fluorescent orange or orange-red with letters or symbols in a contrasting color. These are attached to any container that is used to store or transport potentially infectious materials. (▼ **Figure 3-1**)

Needleless Systems

Needleless systems are available for:

- withdrawal of body fluids after initial venous or arterial access is established

- administration of medications or fluids

- any other procedure involving the potential for an exposure incident for which a needleless system is available as an alternative to the use of needle devices

(▲ **Figure 3-2**)

If needleless systems are not used, needles with engineered sharps injury protection shall be used for:

- withdrawal of body fluids

- accessing a vein or artery

- administration of medications or fluids

- any other procedure involving the potential for an exposure incident for which a needle device with engineered sharps injury protection is available

(▼ **Figure 3-3**)

If sharps other than needle devices are used, these items shall include engineered sharps injury protection.

Evaluating Needleless Systems

There are many new types of needleless systems. Examples of the new types of injection equipment, IV equipment and laboratory equipment include:

- needleguard-sliding sheath/sleeve

- needleguards hinged recap

- needleless jet injection

- retractable needles

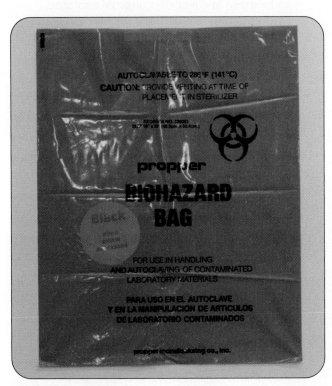

Figure 3-1 Biohazard labels may be attached to bags containing potentially infectious materials. The label must be fluorescent orange or orange-red in color and clearly visible.

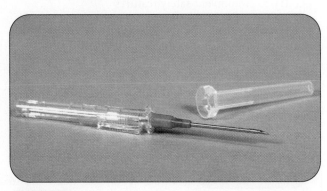

Figure 3-3 IV needle with auto sharp injury protection

- needleless IV access-blunted cannulas
- recessed protected needle
- plastic blood collection tubes
- self-blunting needle
- lancets-laser and retracting
- retracting scalpels
- quick-release scalpel blade handles
- blunted suture needles

If you are stuck by a needle containing blood or OPIM, OSHA recommends:

- an HIV test and counseling
- a test for HIV periodically for at least six months
- practice "safe" sex
- stop breast-feeding
- get immediate evaluation of any illness

You can also call the Needlestick Hotline, which is run by the Department of Health and Human Services and which offers up-to-date, free advice in an emergency 24 hours/day   Telephone: 888-448-4911

Your employer does not have to automatically adopt the most sophisticated engineering controls. They must review and evaluate existing engineering controls and evaluate the feasibility of instituting more advanced methods at your work site.

An example of a safe needle evaluation would be if an employer performed the following steps:

- Determine the product(s) to be evaluated
- Provide a few of each type to each evaluator
- Provide an orange or injection pad to sample the product
- Instruct the evaluators in product use and the product evaluation process
- Encourage comments and suggestions

In turn, the evaluator's role would be to:

- Use the device as you normally would, and
- Try to circumvent safety features

There are many different evaluation forms that can be used. The employer should maintain a file of the forms after they are completed with the action taken regarding the device.

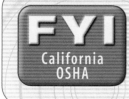

FYI
California
OSHA

CalOSHA's regulation requires that hospitals, physicians, and other health care providers switch to safe needle systems.

Regarding safe needle systems, there are active and passive safety features available. An integrated system is preferred because the safety feature is built in and is not dependent on employee compliance.

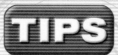

TIPS

According to NIOSH, an estimated 600,000 needle stick injuries occur annually in the hospital setting. Hospital studies reveal that 1/3 of all sharps injuries are related to the disposal process of the sharps.

Engineering Features for Devices Designed to Prevent Sharps Injury

- A fixed safety feature provides a barrier between the hands and the needle after use; the safety feature should allow or require the worker's hands to remain behind the needle at all times.
- The safety feature is an integral part of the device, not an accessory.
- The safety feature is in effect before disassembly and remains in effect after disposal to protect users and trash handlers, and for environmental safety.
- The safety feature is as simple as possible, and requires little or no training to use effectively.

Contaminated Sharps

OSHA defines contaminated sharps as any contaminated object that can penetrate the skin, including, but not limited to, needles, scalpels, broken capillary tubes, and exposed ends of dental wires. (▼ Figure 3-4)

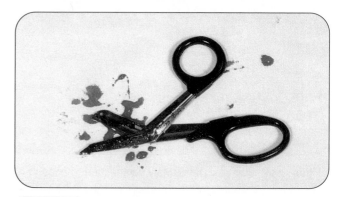

Figure 3-4   Contaminated sharps.

Contaminated needles or other contaminated sharps must not be bent, recapped, or removed unless it can be demonstrated that no alternative is feasible or that such action is required by a specific medical procedure.

If a procedure requires shearing or breaking of needles, this procedure must be specified in the company's Exposure Control Plan. An acceptable means of demonstrating that no alternative to bending, recapping, or removing contaminated needles is feasible or that such action is required by a specific medical procedure would be a written justification (supported by reliable evidence) included as part of the Exposure Control Plan. This justification must state the basis for the determination that no alternative is feasible or must specify that a particular medical procedure requires, for example, the bending of the needle and the use of forceps to accomplish this.

Needle removal or recapping needles must be accomplished through a one-handed technique or the use of a mechanical device. (See Skill Scan on One-Handed Recapping Technique.)

Nurses (RN's and LPN's) were injured more often than any other type of healthcare worker. An overwhelming majority (93%) of the injuries was caused by needles that did not have a safe design. The needles were not shielded, recessed, or retractable.

Reusable Sharps

Reusable sharps must be placed in clearly labeled puncture-resistant, leakproof containers immediately or as soon as possible after use until they can be reprocessed. The containers for reusable sharps are not required to be closable since it is anticipated that containers used for collecting and holding reusable sharps will be reused.

Reusable sharps including pointed scissors that have been contaminated must be decontaminated before reuse. Before cleaning, store the sharps in a container with a wide opening and encourage people to use care in removing items.

Proper decontamination requires all visible blood or OPIM to be rinsed off reusable sharps. Large amounts of organic debris interfere with the efficacy of the disinfecting/sterilization process.

Use a mechanical means (forceps or tongs) to remove contaminated sharps from containers, never reach into any container containing contaminated sharps with your hands. For example, employees must not reach into sinks filled with soapy water into which sharp instruments have been placed; appropriate controls in such a circumstance would include the use of strainer type baskets to hold the instruments and forceps to remove and submerse the items. (▶ Figure 3-5)

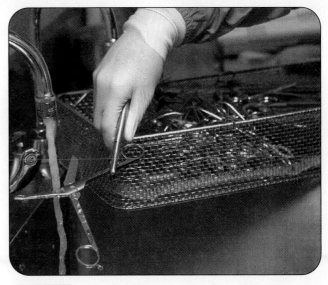

Figure 3-5 Use forceps to remove sharp objects from a strainer.

When it is necessary to examine the contents of a container pour the contents of the container out onto a surface for inspection. An example is inspecting a bag for illegal drugs that might contain a contaminated needle or syringe. The intent is to prevent conditions in which the contents cannot be seen and safely handled.

Acceptable Sharps Containers

The Food and Drug Administration regulate sharps disposal containers as Class II medical devices. OSHA's bloodborne pathogens standard establishes minimum design performance elements for sharps disposal containers. According to the Standard, a sharps container must meet four criteria to be considered acceptable. It must be closable, puncture resistant, leakproof on sides and bottom, and labeled or color-coded in accordance with the Standard. (▼ Figure 3-6)

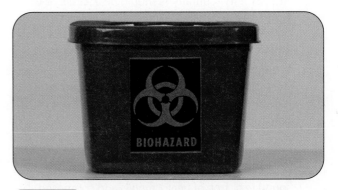

Figure 3-6 Biohazard symbols must be fluorescent orange or orange-red with letters or symbols in a contrasting color. These are attached to any container that is used to store or transport potentially infectious materials.

FDA Classification of Medical Devices

Class I devices (e.g., tongue depressors) are subject only to general regulatory controls and receive little Agency oversight.

Class II devices (e.g., infant incubators) are subject to special controls, such as performance standards, to ensure their safe and effective use.

Class III devices (e.g., implantable pacemakers) are generally life sustaining or life-supporting and are implanted in the body; they present an unreasonable risk of illness of injury.

A sharps container may be made of a variety of products including cardboard or plastic, as long as the four criteria are met. Duct tape may be used to secure a sharps container lid, but it is not acceptable if it serves as the lid itself.

NIOSH criteria for safety performance of sharps containers

1. **Functionality:** Containers should remain **functional** during their entire usage. They should be durable, closable, leak resistant on their sides and bottoms, and puncture resistant until final disposal. A sufficient number of sharps disposal containers should be provided. Individual containers should have adequate volume and safe access to the disposal opening.

2. **Accessibility:** Containers should be **accessible** to workers who use, maintain, or dispose of sharp devices. Containers should be conveniently placed and (if necessary) portable within the workplace.

3. **Visibility:** Containers should be plainly **visible** to the workers who use them. Workers should be able to see the degree to which the container is full, proper warning labels, and color-coding.

4. **Accommodation:** Container designs should be **accommodating** or convenient for the user and the facility, and they should be environmentally sound (e.g., free of heavy metals and composed of recycled materials). **Accommodation** also includes ease of storage and assembly and simplicity of operation.

A sharps container must have a warning label affixed to it. The standard requires that warning labels "be affixed to containers of regulated waste, refrigerators and freezers containing blood or other potentially infectious material; and other containers used to store, transport, or ship blood or other potentially infectious materials."

Using Sharps Containers

Contaminated sharps must be discarded immediately or as soon as feasible into an acceptable sharps container.

Sharps containers must be easily accessible to personnel and located as close as feasible to the immediate area where sharps are used or can be reasonably anticipated to be found. Sharps containers mounted onto walls should be 52" to 56" from the floor.

Sharps containers must be maintained upright throughout use, routinely replaced and not overfilled.

The replacement schedule must be clearly outlined in the Exposure Control Plan. When contaminated sharps are being moved from the area of use it is required that the container be closed immediately prior to removal or replacement to prevent spillage or protrusion of contents during handling, storage, transport, or shipping.

If leakage is possible, or if the outside of the container has become contaminated, the sharps container must be placed in a secondary container that is closable and constructed to contain all contents and prevent leakage during handling, storage, transport, or shipping.

Areas such as correctional facilities, psychiatric units, or pediatric units may have difficulty placing sharps containers in the immediate use area. If workers in these units use a mobile cart to hold the sharps container, it is necessary to lock the sharps container to the cart.

Laundries that handle contaminated laundry must have sharps containers easily accessible due to the incidence of needles mixed with laundry.

Facilities that handle shipments of waste that may contain contaminated sharps must also have sharps containers easily accessible in the event a package accidentally opens and releases sharps.

Finally, the standard requires that reusable containers (such as those used to transport contaminated sharps for cleaning) shall not be opened, emptied, or cleaned manually or in any other manner, which would expose employees to the risk of percutaneous injury.

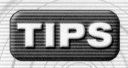 A needle sheath of a self-sheathing needle is not to be considered a "waste container." A self-sheathing needle must be disposed of in a sharps container.

Work Practice Controls

Work practice controls are the behaviors necessary to use engineering controls effectively. These include, but are not limited to, using sharps containers, using an eye wash station, and washing your hands after removing personal protective equipment. An example of a work practice control would be to immediately place contaminated sharps into a sharps container.

All procedures involving blood or OPIM shall be performed in such a way as to minimize or eliminate splashing, spraying, splattering, and generation of droplets of these substances. Not only does this decrease the chances of direct exposure through spraying or splashing of infectious materials onto you, but it also reduces contamination of surfaces in the general work area.

Work practice controls must be evaluated and updated on a regular schedule to ensure their effectiveness.

Mouth pipetting or suctioning of blood or OPIM is prohibited. This procedure should never occur unless it is part of a specialized procedure such as DeLee suctioning. However, even then there must be a one-way valve between the patient and the practitioner.

Eating, drinking, smoking, applying cosmetics or lip balm, and handling contact lenses is prohibited in work areas where there is a reasonable likelihood of occupational exposure to blood or OPIM.

Employees are permitted to eat and drink in an ambulance cab, for example, as long as the employer has implemented procedures to permit employees to wash up and change contaminated clothing prior to entering the ambulance cab, and to ensure that patients and contaminated material remain behind the separating partition.

Hand cream is not considered a cosmetic and is permitted under the standard. It should be noted, however, that some petroleum-based hand creams can adversely affect glove integrity.

Food or drink must not be kept in refrigerators, freezers, shelves, cabinets, countertops, or benches where blood or OPIM is present.

TIPS
Surgical power tools, lasers, and electrocautery devices may generate aerosols as well as be a source for splashing and spattering. Some of these devices include labeling recommendations such as local exhaust ventilation. Your employer is responsible for assuring appropriate operation of these devices, including proper training and use of the controls recommended by the manufacturer.

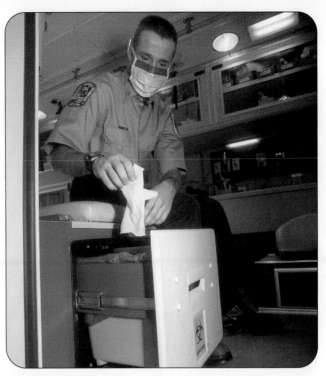

Figure 3-7 Properly dispose of protective equipment in Biohazard containers.

You must remove all personal protective equipment and wash your hands prior to leaving the work area. To prevent contamination of employee eating areas do not enter eating or break areas while wearing personal protective equipment. ▲ **Figure 3-7**

Handwashing and Handwashing Facilities

Handwashing is one of the most effective methods of preventing transmission of bloodborne pathogens. It is required that you wash your hands after removal of gloves and other personal protective equipment. ▼ **Figure 3-8**

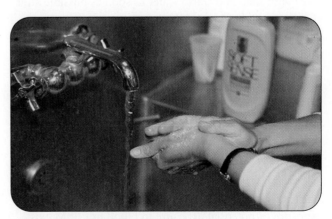

Figure 3-8 Handwashing is a primary means of preventing transmission of bloodborne pathogens.

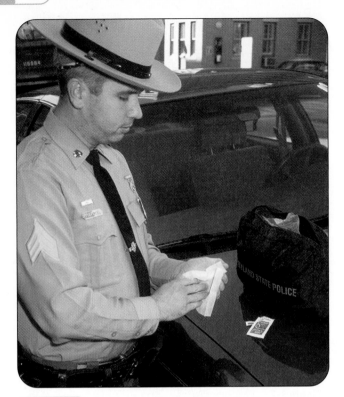

Figure 3-9 Antiseptic wipes can be used when handwashing is not an option.

Employers are required to provide handwashing facilities that are readily accessible to all employees. The standard specifies that the handwashing facility must be situated so that you do not have to use stairs, doorways, and corridors, which might result in environmental surface contamination.

When the provision of handwashing facilities is not feasible (such as in an ambulance or police car), the employer must provide either an appropriate antiseptic hand cleanser with clean cloth or paper towels, or antiseptic towelettes. If you use antiseptic hand cleansers or towelettes, you must wash your hands (or other affected area) with soap and warm water as soon as possible after contact with blood or OPIM. (▲ Figure 3-9)

Employers shall ensure you wash your hands, and any other contaminated skin, with soap and at least tepid running warm water (or flush mucous membranes with water) as soon as possible following contact with blood or OPIM.

Handwashing is required after the removal of gloves because although gloves (vinyl or latex) form a barrier, they are not completely impermeable.

Cleaning Work Surfaces

The term "work area" means the area where work involving exposure or potential exposure to blood or OPIM exists, along with the potential contamination of surfaces.

Groups that may need to use alternative hand washing methods

Groups that may need to use alternative washing methods such as antiseptic hand cleaners and towelettes are ambulance-based paramedics, EMTs, firefighters, police, and mobile blood collection personnel. All employees must wash with soap and warm water as soon as possible after contact with blood or OPIM.

The term "worksite" refers not only to permanent fixed facilities such as hospitals, dental/medical offices, clinics, etc., but also covers temporary non-fixed workplaces. Examples of such facilities include but are not limited to ambulances, bloodmobiles, temporary blood collection centers, and any other non-fixed worksites, which have a reasonable possibility of becoming contaminated with blood or OPIM.

Your employer will identify which work surfaces require inspection for contamination with blood or OPIM and have decontamination on a regularly scheduled basis. This could include, but is not limited to, wastebaskets, exam tables, counters, floors, ambulance interiors, and police cars.

Once a regular inspection and cleaning schedule is established it will need to be followed. The schedule must consider location (exam room versus patient waiting area), type of surface (carpet versus hard floor), type of soil present (gross contamination versus minor splattering), and procedure and tasks performed (laboratory analysis versus patient care). The cleaning schedule must occur at least weekly or after completion of tasks or procedures, after contamination of surfaces, or at the end of a shift if there is a possibility of contamination.

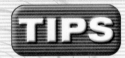

- There is no requirement for handwashing upon leaving the work area unless contact with blood or OPIM has occurred or if you have removed gloves or other PPE.
- Employees must wash hands and skin surfaces after the removal of gloves or other personal protective equipment.
- While extraordinary attempts to disinfect or sterilize environmental surfaces such as walls or floors are rarely indicated, routine cleaning and removal of soil are required.

Receptacles

All bins, pails, cans, and similar receptacles intended for reuse which have a reasonable likelihood for becoming contaminated with blood or OPIM shall be inspected and decontaminated on a regularly scheduled basis and cleaned and decontaminated immediately or as soon as feasible upon visible contamination.

Protective Coverings

Protective coverings, such as plastic wrap, aluminum foil, or imperviously-backed absorbent paper used to cover equipment and environmental surfaces, shall be removed and replaced as soon as feasible when they become overtly contaminated or at the end of the workshift if they may have become contaminated during the shift.

Work Practices

The work surface decontamination is to be performed at the end of the work shift if the work surface may have become contaminated since the last cleaning by, for example, setting down contaminated instruments or specimens on the work surface. This requirement is based upon the existence of a contaminated work surface rather than a particular worksite location. It does not, for example, encompass desks, countertops, and so forth that remain uncontaminated.

Where procedures are performed on a continual basis throughout a shift or a day, as may be the case with a clinical laboratory technician performing blood analyses, it is not necessary for the work surface to be decontaminated before the technician can proceed to the next analysis. Rather, the contaminated work surfaces are to be decontaminated after the procedures are completed which, in the above example, would include a set of analyses. The completion of procedures might also occur when the employee is going to leave the work area for a period of time.

Decontamination Issues

Decontamination is not automatically required after each procedure, but is required only after procedures resulting in surface contamination. There may be some instances in which "immediate" decontamination of overt contamination and spills may not be practical. More stringent decontamination rules, such as cleaning equipment or changing coverings between patients, may be prudent infection control policy but do not fall under OSHA's mandate to safeguard employee (not patient) health.

While cleaning up potentially infectious materials, you must wear reusable medical exam gloves and use an EPA-approved solution. Follow the label instructions regarding the amount of disinfectant and the length of time it must remain wet on the surface. The effectiveness of a disinfectant is governed by strict adherence to the instructions on the label.

Cleansing Solutions

An example of an inexpensive approved solution is 10 percent bleach and water. Fresh solutions of diluted household bleach made up daily (every 24 hours) are also considered appropriate for disinfecting environmental surfaces and for decontamination of sites following initial cleanup of spills of blood or other potentially infectious materials. You should use disposable towels to clean up the spill and then dispose of the towels in a biohazard-labeled bag.

Do not clean up broken glass, that may be contaminated, with your hands. Instead use a dustpan and brush, cardboard, or tongs. The tools, which are used in cleanup (e.g., forceps), must be properly decontaminated or discarded after use. Contaminated broken glass must be placed in a biohazard sharps container. Placing broken glass in a plastic bag may put others at risk for an occupational exposure incident. You must be given specific information and training with respect to this task.

Laundry

Contaminated laundry should be sent to a facility following the OSHA Standard. Your employer must determine if the facility to which laundry is shipped utilizes universal precautions in the handling of all laundry. If not, all bags or containers of contaminated laundry must be labeled or color-coded. The color of the bag **must** be red.

Do not handle laundry any more than necessary. Reducing the amount of manual handling of contaminated laundry reduces the risk of exposure to blood or OPIM and will also reduce contamination of work surfaces in the laundry area.

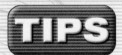

- Hepatitis B Virus (HBV) is able to survive for at least a week in dried blood on environmental surfaces or contaminated instruments.
- Vacuum cleaners are prohibited for the cleaning of broken glass under the Standard.

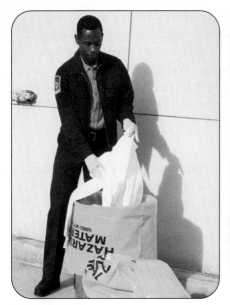

Figure 3-10 Contaminated laundry should be clearly labeled and placed in leakproof containers.

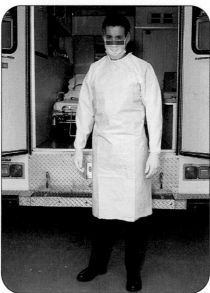

Figure 3-11 Full personal protective equipment includes gloves, gown, mask, and eye shield.

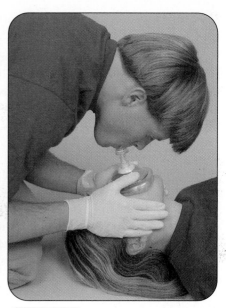

Figure 3-12 Using a pocket mask during CPR prevents exposure to potentially infectious body fluids.

Contaminated laundry should be bagged or placed in an approved container at the location where it was used and shall not be sorted or rinsed in the location of use.

Contaminated laundry shall be placed and transported in bags or containers labeled or color-coded in accordance with the Standard. When a facility utilizes universal precautions in the handling of all soiled laundry, alternative labeling or color-coding is sufficient if it permits all employees to recognize the containers as requiring compliance with universal precautions. **▲ Figure 3-10**

Whenever contaminated laundry is wet and presents a reasonable likelihood of soaking through or leakage from the bag or container, the laundry shall be placed and transported in bags or containers which prevent soak-through and/or leakage of fluids to the exterior.

You must wear protective gloves (e.g., utility gloves) and any other appropriate personal protective equipment, in order to prevent or reduce contact exposure to blood or OPIM when handling laundry or waste materials.

Personal Protective Equipment

Personal protective equipment is specialized clothing or equipment worn or used by you for protection against hazard. This includes equipment such as latex gloves, gowns, aprons, face shields, masks, eye protection, laboratory coats, CPR microshield, and resuscitation bags. PPE prevents blood or OPIM from passing through to, or contacting your work or street clothes, undergarments, skin, eyes, mouth, or other mucous membranes. **▲ Figure 3-11**

Resuscitator devices are to be readily available and accessible to employees who can reasonably be expected to perform resuscitation procedures. Emergency ventilation devices also fall under the scope of PPE and hence must be provided by the employer for use in resuscitation. This includes masks, mouthpieces, resuscitation bags and shields/overlay barriers. **▲ Figure 3-12**

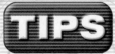

TIPS Home laundering of personal protective equipment is strictly prohibited. Current recommendations for the laundering of contaminated linen stipulate only that normal laundering methods are used according to the manufacturer's recommendations.

Caution:

Do not use a resuscitator device improperly. **It is a violation of the Standard.**

Reasonably anticipated spattering or generation of droplets would necessitate use of eye protection and mask or a face shield to prevent contamination of the mucous membranes of the eyes, nose, and mouth. Whenever you need to wear a face mask, you must also wear eye protection. If you are wearing your personal glasses, you must use side shields and plan to decontaminate your glasses and side shields according to the schedule determined by your employer.

Personal protective equipment is acceptable if it prevents blood or OPIM from contaminating work clothes, street clothes, undergarments, skin, eyes, mouth, or other mucous membranes.

Your employer is responsible for providing personal protective equipment at no expense to you. PPE must be provided in appropriate sizes and placed within easy reach for all employees. Your employer must evaluate the task and the type of exposure expected and, based on the determination, select the "appropriate" personal protective clothing. For example, laboratory coats or gowns with long sleeves must be used for procedures in which exposure of the forearm to blood or OPIM is reasonably anticipated to occur.

Laboratory coats and uniforms that are used as PPE must be laundered by the employer and not sent home with the employee for cleaning. While many employees have traditionally provided and laundered their own uniforms or laboratory coats, if the item's intended function is to act as PPE, then it is your employer's responsibility to provide, clean, repair, replace, and/or dispose of it.

Personal protective equipment, in appropriate sizes and accessible locations, is equipment provided by your employer at no cost to you. Personal protective equipment includes materials such as latex gloves, masks, aprons, gowns, and face shields. It is necessary for you to be trained in the proper use of this equipment. Report to your supervisor when any equipment is not available (e.g. a protective shield is missing) or not in working order (e.g. a hole is in an apron).

You must use personal protective equipment such as gloves or a mask whenever you might be exposed to blood or OPIM.

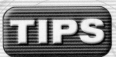
If you choose to wear, and maintain your own uniform or laboratory coat, then you need to don additional employer-handled and employer-controlled PPE when performing tasks where it is reasonable to anticipate exposure to blood or OPIM.

If blood or OPIM contaminates your clothing, you must remove it as soon as feasible and place it in an appropriately designated area or container.

If a pullover scrub or shirt becomes contaminated, you must remove it in such a way as to avoid contact with the outer surface—for example, rolling up the garment as it is pulled toward the head for removal. However, if the blood penetrates the scrub or shirt and contaminates the inner surface, the penetration of the garment itself would constitute an exposure. If the scrub or shirt cannot be removed without contamination of the face, it is recommended that the shirt be cut and removed.

If blood or OPIM has penetrated your personal protective equipment, it is recommended that you check your body for cuts or scrapes or other non-intact skin when removing your equipment. The penetration itself would constitute an exposure of the skin.

You must remove all personal protective equipment before leaving the work area to prevent transmission of bloodborne pathogens to co-workers in other departments and family, and to prevent contamination of environmental surfaces.

Caution:

Do not use PPE improperly. This would include wearing the wrong PPE (e.g., wearing a laboratory coat when a rubber apron is needed) or wearing the wrong size glove.

Gloves

Hypoallergenic gloves, glove liners, powderless gloves, or other similar alternatives must be readily available and accessible at no cost to those employees who are allergic to the gloves normally provided.

The signs and symptoms of latex allergies include skin rashes, inflammation (may be Type I: immediate or Type IV: delayed), respiratory irritation, asthma and in rare cases, shock.

The groups that fall in the high-risk category for latex allergies include healthcare workers and workers in the latex industry.

Latex cross reacts with allergies to certain foods such as avocados, apricots, bananas (most frequent reaction), chestnuts, grapes, kiwi, passion fruit, pears and pineapples.

The occupational issues with latex allergies include more than just the affected employee. Workers with latex sensitivities must use non-latex gloves and their co-workers must use either non-powdered latex or non-latex gloves.

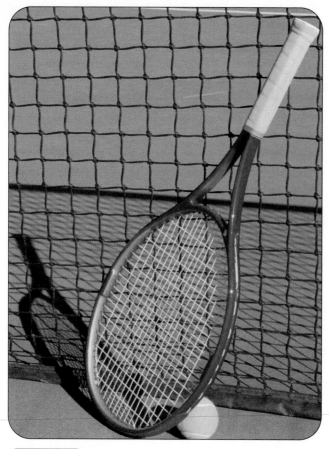

Figure 3-13

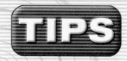

- Studies have shown that gloves provide a barrier, but that neither vinyl nor latex procedure gloves are completely impermeable.

- Disinfecting agents may cause deterioration of the glove material; washing with surfactants could result in wicking or enhanced penetration of liquids into the glove via undetected pores, thereby transporting blood and OPIM into contact with the hand. For this reason, disposable (single-use) gloves may not be washed and reused.

- Certain solutions such as iodine may cause discoloration of gloves without affecting their integrity and function.

Sources of latex exposure can be separated into two categories, medical and household. The following lists outline the possible latex exposures in each of these categories.

Medical

Gloves, urinary catheters, face masks, tourniquet, adhesive tape, bandages, wound drains, injection ports, electrode pads, rubber syringe stoppers and medication vial stoppers, bulb syringes, mattresses on stretchers, dental devices, stethoscopes and blood pressure cuff tubing, ambu bags, PCA syringes and dental dams.

As of 1997, all medical devices containing latex must carry the following statement on the label: "Caution: this product contains natural rubber latex which may cause allergic reactions." As of September 30, 1998, all manufacturing must be in compliance with this law.

Household

Balloons, condoms or diaphragms, rubber bands, shoe soles, erasers, toys, sports equipment, carpet backing, feeding nipples or pacifiers, elastic on underwear, food handled with powdered latex gloves, handles on racquets, tools, diapers, sanitary and incontinence pads, computer mouse pads, and buttons on electronic equipment.

▲ Figure 3-13

Limited Exceptions to Using Personal Protective Equipment

There are a few exceptions to the use of personal protective equipment when the use of such equipment would prevent the proper delivery of healthcare or public safety services, or would pose an increased hazard to the personal safety of the worker. Examples of such situations could include:

- A sudden change in patient status such as when an apparently stable patient unexpectedly begins to hemorrhage profusely, putting the patient's life in immediate jeopardy.

- A firefighter rescuing an individual who is not breathing from a burning building discovers that the resuscitation equipment is lost or damaged and must administer CPR.

- A bleeding suspect unexpectedly attacks a police officer with a knife threatening the safety of the officer and/or co-workers..

Determining the Need for Universal Precautions

Incident	Universal Precautions Needed?	Suggested Action
Nurse is going to change dressing on a recent wound.	YES	Nurse should wear latex gloves and/or personal protective equipment whenever at risk of exposure to blood or potentially infectious materials.
Teacher is approached by young, hysterical student with a bloody nose.	YES	If required to attend to the student, the teacher should reassure child, put on latex gloves and follow routine procedures.
An ambitious attendant is called to a home where an elderly gentleman appears to have had a heart attack. The gentleman is conscious and able to speak.	NO	There is no immediate blood or infectious materials, the attendant may need to perform CPR in the event of cardiac or respiratory arrest. *Note:* In the event of cardiac or respiratory arrest, work practice controls and personal protective equipment may be required.
A police officer pulls over a car that has a burned out headlight.	NO	It is unlikely that the police officer will come in contact with blood or potentially infectious materials.
A laboratory worker is testing urine for evidence of infection. The specimen appears to have a a trace of blood.	YES	The laboratory worker should be using personal protective equipment whenever dealing with any specimens with visible blood.

Universal Precautions

Universal Precautions is an aggressive, standardized approach to infection control. According to the concept of Universal Precautions, you should treat all human blood and certain body fluids as if they are known to contain HIV, HBV, HCV or other bloodborne pathogens, regardless of the perceived risk of the source.

Materials That Require Universal Precautions

Universal Precautions apply to the following potentially infectious materials:

- Blood
- Semen
- Vaginal secretions
- Cerebrospinal fluid
- Synovial fluid
- Pleural fluid
- Any body fluid with visible blood
- Any unidentifiable body fluid
- Saliva from dental procedures

Materials That Do Not Require Universal Precautions

Universal Precautions do not apply to the following body fluids unless they contain visible blood:

- Feces
- Nasal secretions
- Sputum
- Sweat
- Tears
- Urine
- Vomitus

Body Substance Isolation

Another method of infection control is called Body Substance Isolation (BSI). This method defines all body fluids and substances as infectious. BSI includes not only the fluids and other materials covered by this standard, but expands coverage to all body fluids and substances.

BSI is an acceptable alternative to Universal Precautions provided facilities using BSI adhere to all other provisions of this standard.

Skill Scan
One-Handed Recapping Technique

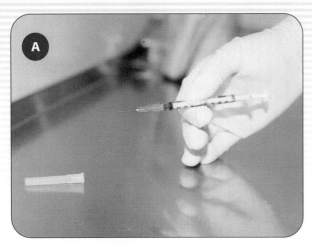

1. Needle removal or recapping must be accomplished through the use of a mechanical device or one-handed technique to prevent puncture wounds.

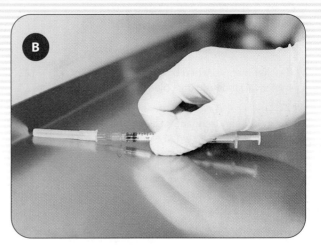

2. Using one hand, gently slide the needle into the needle cover.

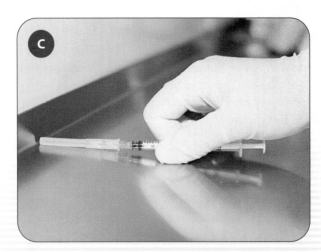

3. Using the wall as support, apply gentle pressure to secure the needle cover.

Skill Scan   Cleaning a Contaminated Spill

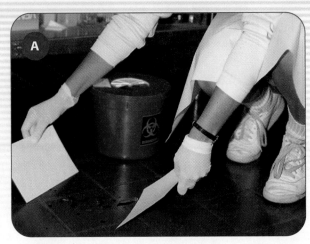

1. When cleaning up broken glass, wear gloves and/or other personal protective equipment.

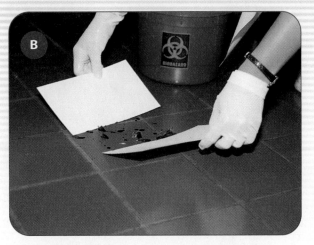

2. Do not clean up broken glass with your hands. Instead use a dust pan and brush, cardboard (as shown), or tongs.

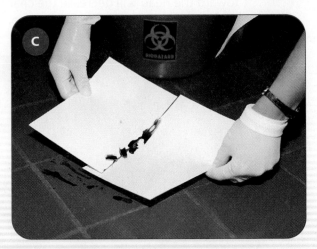

3. Vacuum cleaners are prohibited for the cleaning up of broken glass.

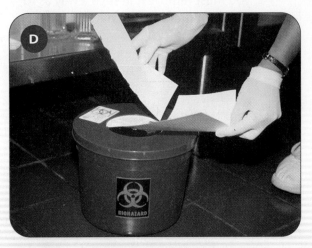

4. Broken glass must be placed in an appropriate sharps container. Placing broken glass in a plastic bag may put others at risk for exposure.

Skill Scan

Removing Contaminated Personal Protective Equipment

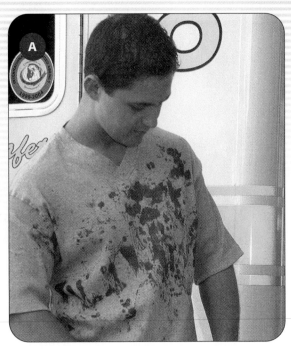

1. If a pull-over shirt becomes contaminated, you must remove it in such a way as to avoid contact with the outer surface.

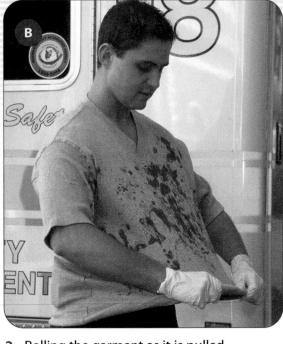

2. Rolling the garment as it is pulled toward the head will decrease the chance of contact with the contaminated area.

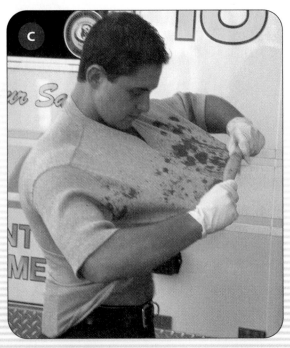

3. After rolling up the shirt, carefully pull it over the head to avoid contact with the face or mucous membranes.

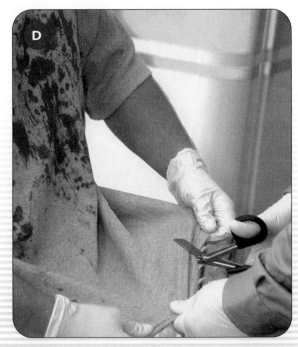

4. If the shirt cannot be removed without contamination, it is recommended that the shirt be cut off.

Site-Specific Work Page

Labeling methods at this worksite include:

color

biohazard symbol (label)

words _____

red bag

The person to notify if you discover regulated waste containers, refrigerators containing blood or OPIM, contaminated equipment, etc. without proper labels is: _____

_____

At my worksite we are expected to adhere to the concept of Universal Precautions. ❏ True ❏ False

According to my employer's Exposure Control Plan, sharps containers are to be inspected every _____

_____

and replaced when: _____

_____

Three examples of engineering controls at my worksite are:

_____

_____

_____

_____

_____

_____

_____

_____

_____

_____

_____

_____

_____

The handwashing station nearest to my worksite is located at: _____

_____

_____

Learning Activities

Yes No   **1.** A gown which is frequently ripped or falls apart under normal use would be considered "appropriate PPE."

T F   **2.** The Exposure Control Plan describes the engineering controls in use at a worksite.

T F   **3.** Duct tape may be used to secure a sharps container lid.

T F   **4.** When cleaning up potentially contaminated broken glass, you may use a dust pan and brush, cardboard or an industrial vacuum cleaner.

T F   **5.** You may launder your own personal protective equipment, but only if this is clearly specified in the Exposure Control Plan.

T F   **6.** Your employer must supply hypoallergenic gloves at no cost to employees who are allergic to the gloves normally provided.

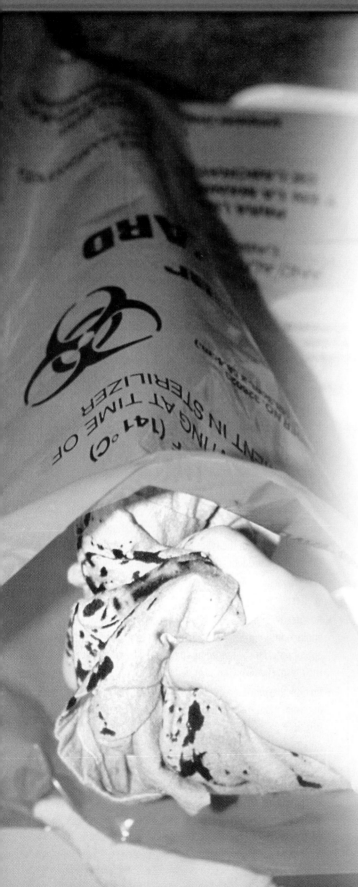

Chapter 4

Exposure Control Plan

Overview

The Exposure Control Plan is a key provision of the OSHA Bloodborne Pathogens Standard. It requires your employer to identify the individuals who receive training, protective equipment, vaccination, and other protections of the standard. The plan must be reviewed annually and updated to reflect significant modifications in tasks or procedures, which may result in occupational exposure to blood or OPIM.

A hard copy of the Exposure Control Plan must be made available to you within 15 working days of your request. This chapter discusses the Exposure Control Plan requirements. A sample "Exposure Control Plan" is included in Appendix C. Please refer to it for guidance relative to compliance with OSHA's Bloodborne Pathogens Standard. (▼ Figure 4-1)

Figure 4-1 All employees must be made aware of an employer's Exposure Control Plan.

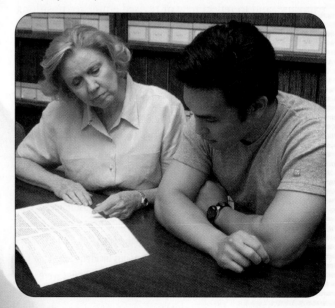

Exposure Control Plan Requirements

The Exposure Control Plan shall contain an exposure determination including:

1. A list of job classifications in which occupational exposure may occur, and/or will occur.

2. Job classifications in which some employees have occupational exposure:

   • The specific tasks and procedures, or groups of closely related tasks and procedures, which are associated with occupational exposure must be delineated. For example, only some of the employees in a hospital laundry room might be assigned the task of handling contaminated laundry.

   • The tasks and procedures that are grouped must be related; i.e., they must share a common activity such as "vascular access procedures," "handling of contaminated sharps," or "handling of deceased persons," etc.

   • The exposure determination must have been made without taking into consideration the use of personal protective clothing or equipment.

The exposure control plan must include the procedure for evaluating the circumstances surrounding exposure incidents. 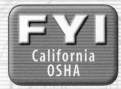 ► Figure 4-2

The Exposure Control Plan shall be reviewed and updated annually and whenever necessary to reflect new or modified tasks and procedures that affect occupational exposure, and to reflect new or revised employee positions with occupational exposure.

The Exposure Control Plan shall be made available to the Assistant Secretary of Labor and the Director on request.

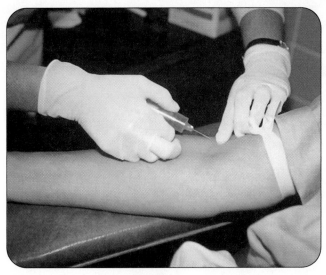

Figure 4-2 All procedures that risk occupational exposure must be outlined in the Exposure Control Plan.

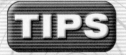

According to the preamble to the standard, the requirement to review and update the plan means that the plan must reflect changes in technology that eliminate or reduce exposure to bloodborne pathogens. The preamble to the Final Rule in 1991 also stated that "with regard to percutaneous incidents, such as needlestick injuries, evidence indicated that most injuries were preventable… 75 percent of all exposure incidents are caused by disposable syringes… and could be prevented by using syringes which incorporate resheathing or retracting designs."

FYI California OSHA

California OSHA adds the following requirements (effective August 1999):

• An effective procedure for gathering the information required by the Sharps Injury Log

• An effective procedure for periodic determination of the frequency of use of the types and brands of sharps involved in the exposure incidents documented on the Sharps Injury Log

NOTE: Frequency of use may be approximated by any reasonable and effective method.

• An effective procedure for identifying currently available engineering controls, and selecting such controls, where appropriate, for the procedures performed by employees in their respective work areas or departments

• An effective procedure for documenting patient safety determinations made pursuant to Exception 2, of subsection (d)(3)(A)

• An effective procedure for obtaining the active involvement of employees in reviewing and updating the exposure control plan with respect to the procedures performed by employees in their respective work areas or departments

• The Exposure Control Plan shall be made available to the Chief of NIOSH or their respective designee upon request for examination and copying

Appendix A

OSHA Bloodborne Pathogens

Regulations Section 1910.1030

Part 1910-[Amended]

Subpart Z-[Amended]

1. The general authority citation for subpart Z of 29 CFR part 1910 continues to read as follows and a new citation for 1910.1030 is added:

Authority: Secs. 6 and 8, Occupational Safety and Health Act, 29 U.S.C. 655, 657, Secretary of Labor's Orders Nos. 12-71 (36 CFR 8754), 8-76 (41 CFR 25059), or 9-83 (48 CFR 35736), as applicable; and 29 CFR part 1911.

*   *   *

Section 1910.1030 also issued under 29 U.S.C. 853.

*   *   *

2. Section 1910.1030 is added to read as follows:

1910.1030 Bloodborne Pathogens.

(a) Scope and Application

This section applies to all occupational exposure to blood or other potentially infectious materials as defined by paragraph (b) of this section.

(b) Definitions

For purposes of this section, the following shall apply:

Assistant Secretary means the Assistant Secretary of Labor for Occupational Safety and Health, or designated representative.

Blood means human blood, human blood components, and products made from human blood.

Bloodborne Pathogens means pathogenic microorganisms that are present in human blood and can cause disease in humans. These pathogens include, but are not limited to, Hepatitis B Virus [HBV] and Human Immunodeficiency Virus [HIV].

Clinical Laboratory means a workplace where diagnostic or other screening procedures are performed on blood or other potentially infectious materials.

Contaminated means the presence or the reasonably anticipated presence of blood or other potentially infectious materials on an item or surface.

Contaminated Laundry means laundry which has been soiled with blood or other potentially infectious materials or may contain sharps.

Contaminated Sharps means any contaminated object that can penetrate the skin including, but not limited to, needles, scalpels, broken glass, broken capillary tubes, and exposed ends of dental wires.

Decontamination means the use of physical or chemical means to remove, inactivate, or destroy bloodborne pathogens on a surface or item to the point where they are no longer capable of transmitting infectious particles and the surface or item is rendered safe for handling, use, or disposal.

Director means the Director of the National Institute for Occupational Safety and Health, U.S. Department of Health and Human Services, or designated representative.

Engineering Controls means controls (e.g., sharps disposal containers, self-sheathing needles) that isolate or remove the bloodborne pathogens hazard from the workplace.

Exposure Incident means a specific eye, mouth, other mucous membrane, non-intact skin, or parenteral contact with blood or other potentially infectious materials that results from the performance of an employee's duties.

Handwashing Facilities means a facility providing an adequate supply of running potable water, soap, and single use towels or hot air drying machines.

Licensed Health Care Professional is a person whose legally permitted scope of practice allows him or her to independently perform the activities required by paragraph (f) Hepatitis B vaccination and Post-Exposure Evaluation and Follow-Up.

HBV means Hepatitis B Virus.

HIV means Human Immunodeficiency Virus.

Occupational Exposure means reasonably anticipated skin, eye, mucous membrane, or parenteral contact with blood or other potentially infectious materials that may result from the performance of an employee's duties.

Other Potentially Infectious Materials means:

(1) The following human body fluids: semen, vaginal secretions, cerebrospinal fluid, synovial fluid, pleural fluid, pericardial fluid, peritoneal fluid, amniotic fluid, saliva in dental procedures, any body fluid that is visibly contaminated with blood, and all body fluids in situations where it is difficult or impossible to differentiate between body fluids;

(2) Any unfixed tissue or organ (other than intact skin) from a human (living or dead); and

(3) HIV-containing cell or tissue cultures, organ cultures, and HIV- or HBV-containing culture medium or other solutions; and blood, organs, or other tissues from experimental animals infected with HIV or HBV.

Parenteral means piercing mucous membranes or the skin barrier through such events as needlesticks, human bites, cuts, and abrasions.

Personal Protective Equipment is specialized clothing or equipment worn by an employee for protection against a hazard. General work clothes (e.g., uniforms, pants, shirts, or blouses) not intended to function as protection against a hazard are not considered to be personal protective equipment.

Production Facility means a facility engaged in industrial-scale, large-volume, or high concentration production of HIV or HBV.

Regulated Waste means liquid or semi-liquid blood or other potentially infectious materials; contaminated items that would release blood or other potentially infectious materials in a liquid or semi-liquid state if compressed; items that are caked with dried blood or other potentially infectious materials and are capable of releasing these materials during handling; contaminated sharps; and pathological and microbiological wastes containing blood or other potentially infectious materials.

Research Laboratory means a laboratory producing or using research-laboratory-scale amounts of HIV or HBV. Research laboratories may produce high concentrations of HIV or HBV but not in the volume found in production facilities.

Source Individual means any individual, living or dead, whose blood or other potentially infectious materials may be a source of occupational exposure to the employee. Examples include, but are not limited to, hospital and clinic patients; clients in institutions for the developmentally disabled; trauma victims; clients of drug and alcohol treatment facilities; residents of hospices and nursing homes; human remains; and individuals who donate or sell blood or blood components.

Sterilize means the use of a physical or chemical procedure to destroy all microbial life including highly resistant bacterial endospores.

Universal Precautions is an approach to infection control. According to the concept of Universal Precautions, all human blood and certain human body fluids are treated as if known to be infectious for HIV, HBV, and other bloodborne pathogens.

Work Practice Controls means controls that reduce the likelihood of exposure by altering the manner in which a task is performed (e.g., prohibiting recapping of needles by a two-handed technique).

(c) Exposure Control

    (1) *Exposure Control Plan.*

        (i)   Each employer having an employee(s) with occupational exposure as defined by paragraph (b) of this section shall establish a written Exposure Control Plan designed to eliminate or minimize employee exposure.

        (ii)   The Exposure Control Plan shall contain at least the following elements:

            (A) The exposure determination required by paragraph (c)(2);

            (B) The schedule and method of implementation for paragraphs (d) Methods of Compliance, (e) HIV and HBV Research Laboratories and Production Facilities, (f) Hepatitis B Vaccination and Post-Exposure Evaluation and Follow-Up, (g) Communication of Hazards to Employees, and (h) Recordkeeping of this standard; and

            (C) The procedure for the evaluation of circumstances surrounding exposure incidents as required by paragraph (f)(3)(i) of this standard.

        (iii) Each employer shall ensure that a copy of the Exposure Control Plan is accessible to employees in accordance with 29 CFR 1910.20(e).

        (iv) The Exposure Control Plan shall be reviewed and updated at least annually and whenever necessary to reflect new or modified tasks and procedures which affect occupational exposure and to reflect new or revised employee positions with occupational exposure.

        (v)   The Exposure Control Plan shall be made available to the Assistant Secretary and the Director upon request for examination and copying.

    (2) *Exposure Determination.*

        (i)   Each employer who has an employee(s) with occupational exposure as defined by paragraph (b) of this section shall prepare an exposure determination. This exposure determination shall contain the following:

            (A) A list of all job classifications in which all employees in those job classifications have occupational exposure;

            (B) A list of job classifications in which some employees have occupational exposure; and

            (C) A list of all tasks and procedures or groups of closely related task and procedures in which occupational exposures occur and that are performed by employees in job classifications listed in accordance with the provisions of paragraph (c)(2)(i)(B) of this standard.

        (ii) This exposure determination shall be made without regard to the use of personal protective equipment.

(d) Methods of Compliance

    (1) *General.*

    Universal precautions shall be observed to prevent contact with blood or other potentially infectious materials. Under circumstances in which differentiation between body fluid types is difficult or impossible, all body fluids shall be considered potentially infectious materials.

    (2) *Engineering and Work Practice Controls.*

        (i)   Engineering and work practice controls shall be used to eliminate or minimize employee exposure. Where occupational exposure remains after institution of these controls, personal protective equipment shall also be used.

        (ii) Engineering controls shall be examined and maintained or replaced on a regular schedule to ensure their effectiveness.

        (iii) Employers shall provide handwashing facilities which are readily accessible to employees.

        (iv) When provision of handwashing facilities is not feasible, the employer shall provide either an appropriate antiseptic hand cleanser in conjunction with clean cloth/paper towels or antiseptic towelettes. When antiseptic hand cleansers or towelettes are used, hands shall be washed with soap and running water as soon as feasible.

        (v)   Employers shall ensure that employees wash their hands immediately or as soon as feasible after removal of gloves or other personal protective equipment.

        (vi) Employers shall ensure that employees wash hands and any other skin with soap and water, or flush mucous membranes with water immediately or as soon as feasible following contact of such body areas with blood or other potentially infectious materials.

(vii) Contaminated needles and other contaminated sharps shall not be bent, recapped, or removed except as noted in paragraphs (d)(2)(vii)(A) and (d)(2)(vii)(B) below. Shearing or breaking of contaminated needles is prohibited.

> (A) Contaminated needles and other contaminated sharps shall not be recapped or removed unless the employer can demonstrate that no alternative is feasible or that such action is required by a specific medical procedure.

> (B) Such recapping or needle removal must be accomplished through the use of a mechanical device or a one-handed technique.

(viii) Immediately or as soon as possible after use, contaminated reusable sharps shall be placed in appropriate containers until properly reprocessed. These containers shall be:

> (A) Puncture resistant;

> (B) Labeled or color-coded in accordance with this standard;

> (C) Leakproof on the sides and bottom; and

> (D) In accordance with the requirements set forth in paragraph (d)(4)(ii)(E) for reusable sharps.

(ix) Eating, drinking, smoking, applying cosmetics or lip balm, and handling contact lenses are prohibited in work areas where there is a reasonable likelihood of occupational exposure.

(x) Food and drink shall not be kept in refrigerators, freezers, shelves, cabinets or on countertops or benchtops where blood or other potentially infectious materials are present.

(xi) All procedures involving blood or other potentially infectious materials shall be performed in such a manner as to minimize splashing, spraying, spattering, and generation of droplets of these substances.

(xii) Mouth pipetting/suctioning of blood or other potentially infectious materials is prohibited.

(xiii) Specimens of blood or other potentially infectious materials shall be placed in a container which prevents leakage during collection, handling, processing, storage, transport, or shipping.

> (A) The container for storage, transport, or shipping shall be labeled or color-coded according to paragraph (g)(1)(i) and closed prior to being stored, transported, or shipped. When a facility utilizes Universal Precautions in the handling of all specimens, the labeling/color-coding of specimens is not necessary provided containers are recognizable as containing specimens. This exemption only applies while such specimens/containers remain within the facility. Labeling or color-coding in accordance with paragraph (g)(1)(i) is required when such specimens/containers leave the facility.

> (B) If outside contamination of the primary container occurs, the primary container shall be placed within a second container which prevents leakage during handling, processing, storage, transport, or shipping and is labeled or color-coded according to the requirements of this standard.

> (C) If the specimen could puncture the primary container, the primary container shall be placed within a secondary container which is puncture-resistant in addition to the above characteristics.

(xiv) Equipment which may become contaminated with blood or other potentially infectious materials shall be examined prior to servicing or shipping and shall be decontaminated as necessary, unless the employer can demonstrate that decontamination of such equipment or portions of such equipment is not feasible.

> (A) A readily observable label in accordance with paragraph (g)(1)(i)(H) shall be attached to the equipment stating which portions remain contaminated.

> (B) The employer shall ensure that this information is conveyed to all affected employees, the servicing representative, and/or the manufacturer, as appropriate, prior to handling, servicing, or shipping so that appropriate precautions will be taken.

(3) *Personal Protective Equipment.*

> (i) Provision. When there is occupational exposure, the employer shall provide, at no cost to the employee, appropriate personal protective equipment such as, but not limited to, gloves, gowns, laboratory coats, face shields or masks and eye protection, and mouthpieces, resuscitation bags, pocket masks, or other ventilation devices. Personal protective equipment will be considered "appropriate" only if it does not permit blood or other potentially infectious materials to pass through to or reach the employee's work clothes, street clothes, undergarments, skin, eyes, mouth, or other mucous membranes under normal conditions of use and for the duration of time which the protective equipment will be used.

> (ii) Use. The employer shall ensure that the employee uses appropriate personal protective equipment unless the employer shows that the employee temporarily and briefly declined to use personal protective equipment when, under rare and extraordinary circumstances, it was the employee's professional judgment that in the specific instance its use would have prevented the delivery of health care or public safety services or would have posed an increased hazard to the safety of the worker or co-worker. When the employee makes this judgment, the circumstances shall be investigated and documented in order to determine whether changes can be instituted to prevent such occurrences in the future.

(iii) Accessibility. The employer shall ensure that appropriate personal protective equipment in the appropriate sizes is readily accessible at the worksite or is issued to employees. Hypoallergenic gloves, glove liners, powderless gloves, or other similar alternatives shall be readily accessible to those employees who are allergic to the gloves normally provided.

(iv) Cleaning, Laundering, and Disposal. The employer shall clean, launder, and dispose of personal protective equipment required by paragraphs (d) and (e) of this standard, at no cost to the employee.

(v) Repair and Replacement. The employer shall repair or replace personal protective equipment as needed to maintain its effectiveness, at no cost to the employee.

(vi) If a garment(s) is penetrated by blood or other potentially infectious materials, the garment(s) shall be removed immediately or as soon as feasible.

(vii) All personal protective equipment shall be removed prior to leaving the work area.

(viii) When personal protective equipment is removed it shall be placed in an appropriately designated area or container for storage, washing, decontamination, or disposal.

(ix) Gloves. Gloves shall be worn when it can be reasonably anticipated that the employee may have hand contact with blood, other potentially infectious materials, mucous membranes, and non-intact skin; when performing vascular access procedures except as specified in paragraph (d)(3)(ix)(D); and when handling or touching contaminated items or surfaces.

(A) Disposable (single-use) gloves such as surgical or examination gloves, shall be replaced as soon as practical when contaminated or as soon as feasible if they are torn, punctured, or when their ability to function as a barrier is compromised.

(B) Disposable (single-use) gloves shall not be washed or decontaminated for re-use.

(C) Utility gloves may be decontaminated for reuse if the integrity of the glove is not compromised. However, they must be discarded if they are cracked, peeling, torn, punctured, or exhibit other signs of deterioration or when their ability to function as a barrier is compromised.

(D) If an employer in a volunteer blood donation center judges that routine gloving for all phlebotomies is not necessary then the employer shall:

(1) Periodically reevaluate this policy;

(2) Make gloves available to all employees who wish to use them for phlebotomy;

(3) Not discourage the use of gloves for phlebotomy; and

(4) Require that gloves be used for phlebotomy in the following circumstances:

(i) When the employee has cuts, scratches, or other breaks in his or her skin;

(ii) When the employee judges that hand contamination with blood may occur, for example, when performing phlebotomy on an uncooperative source individual; and

(iii) When the employee is receiving training in phlebotomy.

(x) Masks, Eye Protection, and Face Shields. Masks in combination with eye protection devices, such as goggles or glasses with solid side shields, or chin-length face shields, shall be worn whenever splashes, spray, spatter, or droplets of blood or other potentially infectious materials may be generated and eye, nose, or mouth contamination can be reasonably anticipated.

(xi) Gowns, Aprons, and Other Protective Body Clothing. Appropriate protective clothing such as, but not limited to, gowns, aprons, lab coats, clinic jackets, or similar outer garments shall be worn in occupational exposure situations. The type and characteristics will depend upon the task and degree of exposure anticipated.

(xii) Surgical caps or hoods and/or shoe covers or boots shall be worn in instances when gross contamination can reasonably be anticipated (e.g., autopsies, orthopedic surgery).

(4) *Housekeeping.*

(i) General. Employers shall ensure that the worksite is maintained in a clean and sanitary condition. The employer shall determine and implement an appropriate written schedule for cleaning and method of decontamination based upon the location within the facility, type of surface to be cleaned, type of soil present, and tasks or procedures being performed in the area.

(ii) All equipment and environmental and working surfaces shall be cleaned and decontaminated after contact with blood or other potentially infectious materials.

(A) Contaminated work surfaces shall be decontaminated with an appropriate disinfectant after completion of procedures; immediately or as soon as feasible when surfaces are overtly contaminated or after any spill of blood or other potentially infectious materials; and at the end of the work shift if the surface may have become contaminated since the last cleaning.

(B) Protective coverings, such as plastic wrap, aluminum foil, or imperviously backed absorbent paper used to cover equipment and environmental surfaces, shall be removed and replaced as soon as feasible when they become overtly contaminated or at the end of the work shift if they may have become contaminated during the shift.

(C) All bins, pails, cans, and similar receptacles intended for reuse which have a reasonable likelihood for becoming contaminated with blood or other potentially infectious materials shall be inspected and decontaminated on a regularly scheduled basis and cleaned and decontaminated immediately or as soon as feasible upon visible contamination.

(D) Broken glassware which may be contaminated shall not be picked up directly with the hands. It shall be cleaned up using mechanical means, such as a brush and dust pan, tongs, or forceps.

(E) Reusable sharps that are contaminated with blood or other potentially infectious materials shall not be stored or processed in a manner that requires employees to reach by hand into the containers where these sharps have been placed.

(iii) Regulated Waste.

(A) Contaminated Sharps Discarding and Containment.

(1) Contaminated sharps shall be discarded immediately or as soon as feasible in containers that are:

(i) Closable;

(ii) Puncture resistant;

(iii) Leakproof on sides and bottom; and

(iv) Labeled or color-coded in accordance with paragraph (g)(1)(i) of this standard.

(2) During use, containers for contaminated sharps shall be:

(i) Easily accessible to personnel and located as close as is feasible to the immediate area where sharps are used or can be reasonably anticipated to be found (e.g., laundries);

(ii) Maintained upright throughout use; and

(iii) Replaced routinely and not be allowed to overfill.

(3) When moving containers of contaminated sharps from the area of use, the containers shall be:

(i) Closed immediately prior to removal or replacement to prevent spillage or protrusion of contents during handling, storage, transport, or shipping;

(ii) Placed in a secondary container if leakage is possible. The second container shall be:

(A) Closable;

(B) Constructed to contain all contents and prevent leakage during handling, storage, transport, or shipping; and

(C) Labeled or color-coded according to paragraph (g)(1)(i) of this standard.

(4) Reusable containers shall not be opened, emptied, or cleaned manually or in any other manner which would expose employees to the risk of percutaneous injury.

(B) Regulated Waste Containment.

(1) Regulated waste shall be placed in containers that are:

(i) Closable;

(ii) Constructed to contain all contents and prevent leakage of fluids during handling, storage, transport, or shipping;

(iii) Labeled or color-coded in accordance with paragraph (g)(1)(i) of this standard; and

(iv) Closed prior to removal to prevent spillage or protrusion of contents during handling, storage, transport, or shipping.

(2) If outside contamination of the regulated waste container occurs, it shall be placed in a second container. The second container shall be:

(i) Closable;

(ii) Constructed to contain all contents and prevent leakage of fluids during handling, storage, transport, or shipping;

(iii) Labeled or color-coded in accordance with paragraph (g)(1)(i) of this standard; and

(iv) Closed prior to removal to prevent spillage or protrusion of contents during handling, storage, transport, or shipping.

(C) Disposal of all regulated waste shall be in accordance with applicable regulations of the United States, States and Territories, and political subdivisions of States and Territories.

(iv) Laundry.

(A) Contaminated laundry shall be handled as little as possible with a minimum of agitation.

(1) Contaminated laundry shall be bagged or containerized at the location where it was used and shall not be sorted or rinsed in the location of use.

(2) Contaminated laundry shall be placed and transported in bags or containers labeled or color-coded in accordance with paragraph (g)(1)(i) of this standard. When a facility utilizes Universal Precautions in the handling of all soiled laundry, alternative labeling or color-coding is sufficient if it permits all employees to recognize the containers as requiring compliance with Universal Precautions.

(3) Whenever contaminated laundry is wet and presents a reasonable likelihood of soak-through of or leakage from the bag or container, the laundry shall be placed and transported in bags or containers which prevent soak-through and/or leakage of fluids to the exterior.

(B) The employer shall ensure that employees who have contact with contaminated laundry wear protective gloves and other appropriate personal protective equipment.

(C) When a facility ships contaminated laundry off-site to a second facility which does not utilize Universal Precautions in the handling of all laundry, the facility generating the contaminated laundry must place such laundry in bags or containers which are labeled or color-coded in accordance with paragraph (g)(1)(i).

(e) HIV and HBV Research Laboratories and Production Facilities.

(1) This paragraph applies to research laboratories and production facilities engaged in the culture, production, concentration, experimentation, and manipulation of HIV and HBV. It does not apply to clinical or diagnostic laboratories engaged solely in the analysis of blood, tissues, or organs. These requirements apply in addition to the other requirements of the standard.

(2) Research laboratories and production facilities shall meet the following criteria:

(i) Standard microbiological practices. All regulated waste shall either be incinerated or decontaminated by a method such as autoclaving known to effectively destroy bloodborne pathogens.

(ii) Special practices:

(A) Laboratory doors shall be kept closed when work involving HIV or HBV is in progress.

(B) Contaminated materials that are to be decontaminated at a site away from the work area shall be placed in a durable, leakproof, labeled or color-coded container that is closed before being removed from the work area.

(C) Access to the work area shall be limited to authorized persons. Written policies and procedures shall be established whereby only persons who have been advised of the potential biohazard, who meet any specific entry requirements, and who comply with all entry and exit procedures shall be allowed to enter the work areas and animal rooms.

(D) When other potentially infectious materials or infected animals are present in the work area or containment module, a hazard warning sign incorporating the universal biohazard symbol shall be posted on all access doors. The hazard warning sign shall comply with paragraph (g)(1)(ii) of this standard.

(E) All activities involving other potentially infectious materials shall be conducted in biological safety cabinets or other physical-containment devices within the containment module. No work with these other potentially infectious materials shall be conducted on the open bench.

(F) Laboratory coats, gowns, smocks, uniforms, or other appropriate protective clothing shall be used in the work area and animal rooms. Protective clothing shall not be worn outside of the work area and shall be decontaminated before being laundered.

(G) Special care shall be taken to avoid skin contact with other potentially infectious materials. Gloves shall be worn when handling infected animals and when making hand contact with other potentially infectious materials is unavoidable.

(H) Before disposal all waste from work areas and from animal rooms shall either be incinerated or decontaminated by a method such as autoclaving known to effectively destroy bloodborne pathogens.

(I) Vacuum lines shall be protected with liquid disinfectant traps and high efficiency particulate air (HEPA) filters or filters of equivalent or superior efficiency and which are checked routinely and maintained or replaced as necessary.

(J) Hypodermic needles and syringes shall be used only for parenteral injection and aspiration of fluids from laboratory animals and diaphragm bottles. Only needle-locking syringes or disposable syringe-needle units (i.e., the needle is integral to the syringe) shall be used for the injection or aspiration of other potentially infectious materials. Extreme caution shall be used when handling needles and syringes. A needle shall not be bent, sheared, replaced in the sheath or guard, or removed from the syringe following use. The needle and syringe shall be promptly placed in a puncture-resistant container and autoclaved or decontaminated before reuse or disposal.

(K) All spills shall be immediately contained and cleaned up by appropriate professional staff or others properly trained and equipped to work with potentially concentrated infectious materials.

(L) A spill or accident that results in an exposure incident shall be immediately reported to the laboratory director or other responsible person.

(M) A biosafety manual shall be prepared or adopted and periodically reviewed and updated at least annually or more often if necessary. Personnel shall be advised of potential hazards, shall be required to read instructions on practices and procedures, and shall be required to follow them.

(iii) Containment Equipment.

(A) Certified biological safety cabinets (Class II, III, or IV) or other appropriate combinations of personal protection or physical containment devices, such as special protective clothing, respirators, centrifuge safety cups, sealed centrifuge rotors, and containment caging for animals, shall be used for all activities with other potentially infectious materials that pose a threat of exposure to droplets, splashes, spills, or aerosols.

(B) Biological safety cabinets shall be certified when installed, whenever they are moved, and at least annually.

(3) HIV and HBV research laboratories shall meet the following criteria:

(i) Each laboratory shall contain a facility for handwashing and an eye wash facility which is readily available within the work area.

(ii) An autoclave for decontamination or regulated waste shall be available.

(4) HIV and HBV production facilities shall meet the following criteria:

(i) The work areas shall be separated from areas that are open to unrestricted traffic flow within the building. Passage through two sets of doors shall be the basic requirement for entry into the work area from access corridors or other contiguous areas. Physical separation of the high-containment work area from access corridors or other areas or activities may also be provided by a double-doored clothes-change room (showers may be included), airlock, or other access facility that requires passing through two sets of doors before entering the work area.

(ii) The surfaces of doors, walls, floors, and ceilings in the work area shall be water resistant so that they can be easily cleaned. Penetrations in these surfaces shall be sealed or capable of being sealed to facilitate decontamination.

(iii) Each work area shall contain a sink for washing hands and readily available eye wash facility. The sink shall be foot, elbow, or automatically operated and shall be located near the exit door of the work area.

(iv) Access doors to the work area or containment module shall be self-closing.

(v) An autoclave for decontamination of regulated waste shall be available within or as near as possible to the work area.

(vi) A ducted exhaust-air ventilation system shall be provided. This system shall create directional airflow that draws air into the work area through the entry area. The exhaust air shall not be recirculated to any other area of the building, shall be discharged to the outside, and shall be dispersed away from occupied areas and air intakes. The proper direction of the airflow shall be verified (i.e., into the work area).

(5) *Training Requirements.*

Additional training requirements for employees in HIV and HBV research laboratories and HIV and HBV production facilities are specified in paragraph (g)(2)(ix).

(f) Hepatitis B Vaccination and Post-Exposure Evaluation and Follow-Up.

(1) *General.*

(i) The employer shall make available the Hepatitis B vaccine and vaccination series to all employees who have occupational exposure, and post-exposure evaluation and follow-up to all employees who have had an exposure incident.

(ii) The employer shall ensure that all medical evaluations and procedures including the Hepatitis B vaccine and vaccination series and post-exposure evaluation and follow-up, including prophylaxis, are:

(A) Made available at no cost to the employee;

(B) Made available to the employee at a reasonable time and place;

(C) Performed by or under the supervision of a licensed physician or by or under the supervision of another licensed health care professional; and

(D) Provided according to recommendations of the U.S. Public Health Service current at the time these evaluations and procedures take place, except as specified by this paragraph (f).

(iii) The employer shall ensure that all laboratory tests are conducted by an accredited laboratory at no cost to the employee.

(2) *Hepatitis B Vaccination.*

(i) Hepatitis B vaccination shall be made available after the employee has received the training required in paragraph (g)(2)(vii)(I) and within 10 working days of initial assignment to all employees who have occupational exposure unless the employee has previously received the complete Hepatitis B vaccination series, antibody testing has revealed that the employee is immune, or the vaccine is contraindicated for medical reasons.

(ii) The employer shall not make participation in a prescreening program a prerequisite for receiving Hepatitis B vaccination.

(iii) If the employee initially declines Hepatitis B vaccination but at a later date while still covered under the standard decides to accept the vaccination, the employer shall make available Hepatitis B vaccination at that time.

(iv) The employer shall assure that employees who decline to accept Hepatitis B vaccination offered by the employer sign the statement in Appendix A.

(v) If a routine booster dose(s) of Hepatitis B vaccine is recommended by the U.S. Public Health Service at a future date, such booster dose(s) shall be made available in accordance with section (f)(1)(ii).

(3) *Post-Exposure Evaluation and Follow-Up.*

Following a report of an exposure incident, the employer shall make immediately available to the exposed employee a confidential medical evaluation and follow-up, including at least the following elements:

(i) Documentation of the route(s) of exposure, and the circumstances under which the exposure incident occurred;

(ii) Identification and documentation of the source individual, unless the employer can establish that identification is infeasible or prohibited by state or local law:

(A) The source individual's blood shall be tested as soon as feasible and after consent is obtained in order to determine HBV and HIV infectivity. If consent is not obtained, the employer shall establish that legally required consent cannot be obtained. When the source individual's consent is not required by law, the source individual's blood, if available, shall be tested and the results documented.

(B) When the source individual is already known to be infected with HBV or HIV, testing for the source individual's known HBV or HIV status need not be repeated.

(C) Results of the source individual's testing shall be made available to the exposed employee, and the employee shall be informed of applicable laws and regulations concerning disclosure of the identity and infectious status of the source individual.

(iii) Collection and testing of blood for HBV and HIV serological status:

(A) The exposed employee's blood shall be collected as soon as feasible and tested after consent is obtained.

(B) If the employee consents to baseline blood collection, but does not give consent at that time for HIV serologic testing, the sample shall be preserved for at least 90 days. If, within 90 days of the exposure incident, the employee elects to have the baseline sample tested, such testing shall be done as soon as feasible.

(iv) Post-exposure prophylaxis, when medically indicated, as recommended by the U.S. Public Health Service;

(v) Counseling; and

(vi) Evaluation of reported illnesses.

(4) *Information Provided to the Health Care Professional.*

(i) The employer shall ensure that the health care professional responsible for the employee's Hepatitis B vaccination is provided a copy of this regulation.

(ii) The employer shall ensure that the health care professional evaluating an employee after an exposure incident is provided the following information:

(A) A copy of this regulation;

(B) A description of the exposed employee's duties as they relate to the exposure incident;

(C) Documentation of the route(s) of exposure and circumstances under which the exposure occurred;

(D) Results of the source individual's blood testing, if available; and

(E) All medical records relevant to the appropriate treatment of the employee including vaccination status which are the employer's responsibility to maintain.

(5) *Health Care Professional's Written Opinion.*

The employer shall obtain and provide the employee with a copy of the evaluating health care professional's written opinion within 15 days of the completion of the evaluation.

(i) The health care professional's written opinion for Hepatitis B vaccination shall be limited to whether Hepatitis B vaccination is indicated for an employee, and if the employee has received such vaccination.

(ii) The health care professional's written opinion for post-exposure evaluation and follow-up shall be limited to the following information:

(A) That the employee has been informed of the results of the evaluation; and

(B) That the employee has been told about any medical conditions resulting from exposure to blood or other potentially infectious materials which require further evaluation or treatment.

(iii) All other findings or diagnoses shall remain confidential and shall not be included in the written report.

(6) *Medical Recordkeeping.*

Medical records required by this standard shall be maintained in accordance with paragraph (h)(1) of this section.

(g) *Communication of Hazards to Employees.*

(1) *Labels and Signs*

(i) Labels

(A) Warning labels shall be affixed to containers of regulated waste, refrigerators and freezers containing blood or other potentially infectious material; and other containers used to store, transport, or ship blood or other potentially infectious materials, except as provided in paragraph (g)(1)(i)(E), (F), and (G).

(B) Labels required by this section shall include the BIOHAZARD legend:

BIOHAZARD

(C) These labels shall be fluorescent orange or orange-red or predominantly so, with lettering or symbols in contrasting color.

(D) Labels required by affixed as close as feasible to the container by string, wire, adhesive, or other method that prevents their loss or unintentional removal.

(E) Red bags or red containers may be substituted for labels.

(F) Containers of blood, blood components, or blood products that are labeled as to their contents and have been released for transfusion or other clinical use are exempted from labeling requirements of paragraph (g).

(G) Individual containers of blood or other potentially infectious materials that are placed in a labeled container during storage, transport, shipment, or disposal are exempted from the labeling requirement.

(H) Labels required for contaminated equipment shall be in accordance with this paragraph and shall also state which portions of the equipment remain contaminated.

(I) Regulated waste that has been decontaminated need not be labeled or color-coded.

(ii) Signs.

(A) The employer shall post signs at the entrance to work areas specified in paragraph (e), HIV and HBV Research Laboratory and Production Facilities, which shall bear the [BIOHAZARD] legend.

BIOHAZARD

(Name of the Infectious Agent)
(Special requirements for entering the area)
(Name, telephone number of the laboratory director or other responsible person)

(B) These signs shall be fluorescent orange-red or predominantly so, with lettering or symbols in a contrasting color.

(2) *Information and Training.*

(i) Employers shall ensure that all employees with occupational exposure participate in a training program which must be provided at no cost to the employee and during working hours.

(ii) Training shall be provided as follows:

(A) At the time of initial assignment to tasks where occupational exposure may take place;

(B) Within 90 days after the effective date of the standard; and

(C) At least annually thereafter.

(iii) For employees who have received training on bloodborne pathogens in the year preceding the effective date of the standard, only training with respect to the provisions of the standard which were not included need be provided.

(iv) Annual training for all employees shall be provided within one year of their previous training.

(v) Employers shall provide additional training when changes such as modification of tasks or procedures or institution of new tasks or procedures affect the employee's occupational exposure. The additional training may be limited to addressing the new exposures created.

(vi) Material appropriate in content and vocabulary to educational level, literacy, and language of employees shall be used.

(vii) The training program shall contain at a minimum the following elements:

(A) An accessible copy of the regulatory text of this standard and an explanation of its contents;

(B) A general explanation of the epidemiology and symptoms of bloodborne diseases;

(C) An explanation of the modes of transmission of bloodborne pathogens;

(D) An explanation of the employer's exposure control plan and the means by which the employee can obtain a copy of the written plan;

(E) An explanation of the appropriate methods for recognizing tasks and other activities that may involve exposure to blood and other potentially infectious materials;

(F) An explanation of the use and limitations of methods that will prevent or reduce exposure including appropriate engineering controls, work practices, and personal protective equipment;

(G) Information on the types, proper use, location, removal, handling, decontamination, and disposal of personal protective equipment;

(H) An explanation of the basis for selection of personal protective equipment;

(I) Information on the Hepatitis B vaccine, including information on its efficacy, safety, method of administration, the benefits of being vaccinated, and that the vaccine and vaccination will be offered free of charge;

(J) Information on the appropriate actions to take and persons to contact in an emergency involving blood or other potentially infectious materials;

(K) An explanation of the procedure to follow if an exposure incident occurs, including the method of reporting the incident and the medical follow-up that will be made available;

(L) Information on the post-exposure evaluation and follow-up that the employer is required to provide for the employee following an exposure incident;

(M) An explanation of the signs and labels and/or color-coding required by paragraph (g)(1); and

(N) An opportunity for interactive questions and answers with the person conducting the training session.

(viii) The person conducting the training shall be knowledgeable in the subject matter covered by the elements contained in the training program as it relates to the workplace that the training will address.

(ix) Additional Initial Training for Employees in HIV and HBV Laboratories and Production Facilities. Employees in HIV or HBV research laboratories and HIV or HBV production facilities shall receive the following initial training in addition to the above training requirements:

(A) The employer shall assure that employees demonstrate proficiency in standard micro-biological practices and techniques and in the practices and operations specific to the facility before being allowed to work with HIV or HBV.

(B) The employer shall assure that employees have prior experience in the handling of human pathogens or tissue cultures before working with HIV or HBV.

(C) The employer shall provide a training program to employees who have no prior experience in handling human pathogens. Initial work activities shall not include the handling of infectious agents. A progression of work activities shall be assigned as techniques are learned and proficiency is developed. The employer shall assure that employees participate in work activities involving infectious agents only after proficiency has been demonstrated.

(h) Recordkeeping.

(1) *Medical Records*

(i) The employer shall establish and maintain an accurate record for each employee with occupational exposure, in accordance with 29 CFR 1910.20.

(ii) This record shall include:

(A) The name and social security number of the employee;

(B) A copy of the employee's Hepatitis B vaccination status including the dates of all the Hepatitis B vaccinations and any medical records relative to the employee's ability to receive vaccination as required by paragraph (f)(2);

(C) A copy of all results of examinations, medical testing, and follow-up procedures as required by paragraph (f)(3);

(D) The employer's copy of the health care professional's written opinion as required by paragraph (f)(5); and

(E) A copy of the information provided to the health care professional as required by paragraphs (f)(4)(ii)(B), (C), and (D).

(iii) Confidentiality. The employer shall ensure that employee medical records required by paragraph (h)(1) are:

(A) Kept confidential; and

(B) Not disclosed or reported without the employee's express written consent to any person within or outside the workplace except as required by this section or as may be required by law.

(iv) The employer shall maintain the records required by paragraph (h) for at least the duration of employment plus 30 years in accordance with 29 CFR 1910.20.

(2) *Training Records*

(i) Training records shall include the following information:

(A) The dates of the training sessions;

(B) The contents or a summary of the training sessions;

(C) The names and qualifications for the persons conducting the training; and

(D) The names and job titles of all persons attending the training sessions.

(ii) Training records shall be maintained for 3 years from the date on which the training occurred.

(3) *Availability*

(i) The employer shall ensure that all records required to be maintained by this section shall be made available upon request to the Assistant Secretary and Director for examination and copying.

(ii) Employee training records required by this paragraph shall be provided upon request for examination and copying to employees, to employee representatives, to the Director, and to the Assistant Secretary in accordance with 29 CFR 1910.20.

(iii) Employee medical records required by this paragraph shall be provided upon request for examination and copying to the subject employee, to anyone having written consent of the subject employee, to the Director, and to the Assistant Secretary in accordance with 29 CFR 1910.20

(4) *Transfer of Records*

(i) The employer shall comply with the requirements involving transfer of records set forth in 29 CFR 1910.20(h).

(ii) If the employer ceases to do business and there is no successor employer to receive and retain the records for the prescribed period, the employer shall notify the Director, at least three months prior to their disposal and transmit them to the Director, if required by the Director to do so, within that three month period.

(i) Dates.

(1) *Effective Date.* The standard shall become effective on March 6, 1992.

(2) The Exposure Control Plan required by paragraph (c)(1) of this section shall be completed on or before May 5, 1992.

(3) Paragraph (g)(2) Information and Training and (h) Recordkeeping shall take effect on or before June 4, 1992.

(4) Paragraphs (d)(2) Engineering and Work Practice Controls, (d)(3) Personal Protective Equipment, (d)(4), Housekeeping, (e) HIV and HBV Research Laboratories and Production Facilities, (f) Hepatitis B Vaccination and Post-Exposure Evaluation and Follow-Up, and (g)(1) Labels and Signs shall take effect July 6, 1992.

Appendix A to Section 1910.1030—

Hepatitis B Vaccine Declination (Mandatory)

I understand that due to my occupational exposure to blood or other potentially infectious materials I may be at risk of acquiring Hepatitis B Virus (HBV) infection. I have been given the opportunity to be vaccinated with Hepatitis B vaccine, at no charge to myself. However, I decline Hepatitis B vaccination at this time. I understand that by declining this vaccine, I continue to be at risk of acquiring Hepatitis B, a serious disease. If in the future I continue to have occupational exposure to blood or other potentially infectious materials and I want to be vaccinated with Hepatitis B vaccine, I can receive the vaccination series at no charge to me.

Appendix B

Hepatitis B Vaccine Declination Form

Appendix A to Section 1910.1030—
Hepatitis B Vaccine Declination (Mandatory)

I understand that due to my occupational exposure to blood or other potentially infectious materials I may be at risk of acquiring Hepatitis B Virus (HBV) infection. I have been given the opportunity to be vaccinated with Hepatitis B vaccine, at no charge to myself. However, I decline the Hepatitis B vaccination at this time. I understand that by declining this vaccine, I continue to be at risk of acquiring Hepatitis B, a serious disease. If in the future I continue to have occupational exposure to blood or other potentially infectious materials and I want to be vaccinated with Hepatitis B vaccine, I can receive the vaccination series at no charge to me.

Employee Signature _____

Date _____

Employer Signature _____

Date _____

Appendix C

Sample Exposure Control Plan

This sample plan is provided as a guide to assist in complying with 29 CFR 1910.1030, OSHA's Bloodborne Pathogens Standard. It is not intended to supersede the requirements detailed in the standard. Employers should review the standard for particular requirements which are applicable to their specific situation. It should be noted that this model program does not include provisions for HIV/ HBV laboratories and research facilities which are addressed in section (e) of the standard. Employers operating these laboratories need to include provisions as required by the standard. Employers will need to add information relevant to their particular facility in order to develop an effective, comprehensive exposure control plan. Employers should note that the exposure control plan is expected to be reviewed at least on an annual basis and updated when necessary.

Bloodborne Pathogens Exposure Control Plan

Facility Name: _____

Date of Preparation: _____

Program Administration

(Name of responsible person or department) is (are) responsible for the implementation of the ECP. **(Name of responsible person or department)** will maintain, review, and update the ECP at least annually, and whenever necessary to include new or modified tasks and procedures. Contact location/phone number: _____

Those employees who are determined to have occupational exposure to blood or other potentially infectious materials (OPIM) must comply with the procedures and work practices outlined in this ECP.

(Name of responsible person or department) will maintain and provide all necessary personal protective equipment (PPE), engineering controls (e.g., sharps containers), labels, and red bags as required by the standard. **(Name of responsible person or department)** will ensure that adequate supplies of the aforementioned equipment are available in the appropriate sizes. Contact location/phone number: _____

(Name of responsible person or department) will be responsible for ensuring that all medical actions required are performed and that appropriate employee health and OSHA records are maintained. Contact location/phone number: _____

(Name of responsible person or department) will be responsible for training, documentation of training, and making the written ECP available to employees, OSHA, and NIOSH representatives. Contact location/phone number: _____

Exposure Control Plan

Employees covered by the bloodborne pathogens standard receive an explanation of this ECP during their initial training session. It will also be reviewed in their annual refresher training. All employees have an opportunity to review this plan at any time during their work shifts by contacting **(Name of responsible person or department)**. If requested, we will provide an employee with a copy of the ECP free of charge and within 15 days of the request.

(Name of responsible person or department) is responsible for reviewing and updating the ECP annually or more frequently if necessary to reflect any new or modified tasks and procedures which affect occupational exposure and to reflect new or revised employee positions with occupational exposure.

In accordance with the OSHA Bloodborne Pathogens Standard, 29 CFR 1910.1030, the following Exposure Control Plan has been developed:

1. Exposure Determination

OSHA requires employers to perform an exposure determination concerning which employees may incur occupational exposure to blood or other potentially infectious materials. The exposure determination is made without regard to the use of personal protective equipment (i.e., employees are considered to be exposed even if they wear personal protective equipment). This exposure determination is required to list all job classifications in which all employees may be expected to incur such occupational exposure, regardless of frequency. At this facility the following job classifications are in this category:

In addition, OSHA requires a listing of job classifications in which some employees may have occupational exposure. Because not all the employees in these categories would be expected to incur exposure to blood or other potentially infectious materials, tasks or procedures that would cause these employees to have occupational exposure must also be listed in order to understand clearly which employees in these categories are considered to have occupational exposure. The job classifications and associated tasks for these categories are as follows:

Job Classification   *Tasks/Procedures*

_____   _____

_____   _____

_____   _____

2. Implementation Schedule and Methodology

OSHA also requires that this plan include a schedule and method of implementation for the various requirements of the standard. The following complies with this requirement:

Compliance Methods

Universal Precautions will be observed at this facility in order to prevent contact with blood or other potentially infectious materials. All blood or other potentially infectious material will be considered infectious regardless of the perceived status of the source individual.

Engineering and work practice controls will be used to eliminate or minimize exposure to employees at this facility. Where occupational exposure remains after institution of these controls, personal protective equipment shall also be used. At this facility the following engineering controls will be used: (list controls, such as sharps containers, etc.).

The above controls will be examined and maintained on a regular schedule. The schedule for reviewing the effectiveness of the controls is as follows: (list schedule such as daily, once/week, etc., as well as who is responsible for reviewing the effectiveness of the individual controls, such as the supervisor for each department, etc.).

Handwashing facilities are also available to the employees who incur exposure to blood or other potentially infectious materials. OSHA requires that these facilities be readily accessible after incurring exposure. At this facility hand-washing facilities are located: (list locations, such as patient rooms, procedure area, etc. If handwashing facilities are not feasible, the employer is required to provide either an anti-septic cleanser in conjunction with a clean cloth/paper towels or antiseptic towelettes. If these alternatives are used then the hands are to be washed with soap and running water as soon as feasible.

Employers who must provide an alternative to readily accessible handwashing facilities should list the location, tasks, and responsibilities to ensure maintenance and accessibility or these alternatives).

After removal of personal protective gloves, employees shall wash hands and any other potentially contaminated skin area immediately or as soon as feasible with soap and water.

If employees incur exposure to their skin or mucous membranes then those areas shall be washed or flushed with water as appropriate as soon as feasible following contact.

Needles

Contaminated needles and other contaminated sharps will not be bent, recapped, removed, sheared, or purposely broken. OSHA allows an exception to this if the procedure would require that the contaminated needles be recapped or removed and no alternative is feasible and the action is required by the medical procedure. If such action is required then the recapping or removal of the needle must be done by the use of a mechanical device or a one-handed technique. At this facility recapping or removal is only permitted for the following procedures: (list the procedures and also list either the mechanical device to be used or alternatively if a one-handed technique will be used).

Containers for Reusable Sharps

Contaminated sharps that are reusable are to be place immediately, or as soon as possible, after use into appropriate sharps containers. At this facility the sharps containers are puncture resistant, labeled with a biohazard label, and are leakproof. (Employers should list here where sharps container are located as well as who has responsibility for removing sharps from containers and how often the containers will be checked to remove the sharps.)

Work Area Restrictions

In work areas where there is a reasonable likelihood of exposure to blood or other potentially infectious materials, employees are not to eat, drink, apply cosmetics or lip balm, smoke, or handle contact lenses. Food and beverages are not to be kept in refrigerators, freezers, shelves, cabinets, or on countertops or benchtops where blood or other potentially infectious materials are present.

Mouth pipetting/suctioning of blood or other potentially infectious materials is prohibited.

All procedures will be conducted in a manner that will minimize splashing, spraying, splattering, and generation of droplets of blood or other potentially infectious materials. Methods to accomplish this goal at this facility are: (list methods, such as covers on centrifuges, usage of dental dams if appropriate, etc.).

Specimens

Specimens of blood or other potentially infectious materials will be placed in a container that prevents leakage during the collection, handling, processing, storage, and transport of the specimens.

The container used for this purpose will be labeled or color-coded in accordance with the requirements of the OSHA standard. (Employers should note that the standard provides for an exemption for specimens from the labeling/color-coding requirement of the standard provided that the facility uses Universal Precautions in the handling of all specimens and the containers are recognizable as container specimens. This exemption applies only while the specimens remain in the facility. If the employer chooses to use this exemption then it should be stated here.)

Any specimens that could puncture a primary container will be placed within a puncture-resistant secondary container. (The employer should list here how this will be carried out, e.g., which specimens, if any, could puncture a primary container, which containers can be used as secondary containers, and where the secondary containers are located at the facility.)

If outside contamination of the primary container occurs, the primary container shall be placed within a secondary container that prevents leakage during the handling, processing, storage, transport, or shipping of the specimen.

Contaminated Equipment

Equipment that has become contaminated with blood or other potentially infectious materials shall be examined before servicing or shipping and shall be decontaminated as necessary unless the decontamination of the equipment is not feasible. (Employers should list here any equipment that cannot be decontaminated before servicing or shipping.)

Personal Protective Equipment

All personal protective equipment used at this facility will be provided without cost to employees. Personal protective equipment will be chosen based on the anticipated exposure to blood or other potentially infectious materials. The protective equipment will be considered appropriate only if it does not permit blood or other potentially infectious materials to pass through or reach the employees' clothing, skin, eyes, mouth, or other mucous membranes under normal conditions of use and for the duration of time that the protective equipment will be used.

Protective clothing will be provided to employees in the following manner: (list how the clothing will be provided to employees, e.g., who has responsibility for distribution, etc., and also list which procedures would require the protective clothing and the type of protections required. This could also be listed as an appendix to this program. The employer could use a checklist as follows):

Personal Protective Equipment	Task
❑ Gloves	_____
❑ Lab coat	_____
❑ Face shield	_____
❑ Clinic jacket	_____
❑ Protective eyewear (with solid side shield)	_____
❑ Surgical gown	_____
❑ Shoe covers	_____
❑ Utility gloves	_____
❑ Examination gloves	_____
❑ Other (list other personal protective equipment)	_____

All personal protective equipment will be cleaned, laundered, and disposed of by the employer at no cost to employees. All repairs and replacements will be made by the employer at no cost to employees.

All garments that are penetrated by blood shall be removed immediately or as soon as feasible. All personal protective equipment will be removed before leaving the work area. The following protocol has been developed to facilitate leaving the equipment at the work area: (list where employees are expected to place the personal protective equipment on leaving the work area, and other protocols).

Gloves shall be worn where it is reasonably anticipated that employees will have hand contact with blood, other potentially infectious materials, non-intact skin, and mucous membranes. Gloves will be available from (state location and/or person who will be responsible for distributing gloves). Gloves will be used for the following procedures: (list procedures).

Disposable gloves used at the facility are not to be washed or decontaminated for re-use and are to be replaced as soon as practical when they become contaminated or as soon as feasible if they are torn, punctured, or when their ability to function as a barrier is compromised. Utility gloves may be decontaminated for re-use provided that the integrity of the glove is not compromised. Utility gloves will be discarded if they are cracked, peeling, torn, punctured, or exhibit other signs of deterioration or when their ability to function as a barrier is compromised.

Masks in combination with eye protection devices, such as goggles or glasses with solid side shield, or chin-length face shield, are required to be worn whenever splashes, spray, splatter, or droplets of blood or other potentially infectious materials may be generated and eye, nose, or mouth contamination can reasonably be anticipated. Situations at this facility that would require such protection are as follows:

The OSHA standard also requires appropriate protective clothing to be used, such as lab coats, gowns, aprons, clinic jackets, or similar outer garments. The following situations require that such protective clothing be worn:

Housekeeping

This facility will be cleaned and decontaminated according to the following schedule: (list area and time).

Decontamination will be accomplished by using the following materials: (list the materials to be used, such as bleach solutions or EPA-registered germicides).

All contaminated work surfaces will be decontaminated after completion of procedures, immediately or as soon as feasible after any spill of blood or other potentially infectious materials, as well as at the end of the work shift if surfaces may have become contaminated since the last cleaning. (Employers should add any information concerning the use of protective coverings such as plastic wrap that keeps the surfaces free of contamination.)

All bins, pails, cans, and similar receptacles shall be inspected and decontaminated on a regularly scheduled basis (list frequency and by whom).

Any broken glassware that may be contaminated will not be picked up directly with the hands. The following procedures will be used: _____

Labels

The following labeling method(s) is/are used in this facility:

EQUIPMENT TO BE LABELED	LABEL TYPE (size, color, etc.)
_____	_____
_____	_____

(Name of responsible person or department) will ensure warning labels are affixed or red bags are used as required if regulated waste or contaminated equipment is brought into the facility. Employees are to notify _____ if they discover regulated waste containers, refrigerators containing blood or OPIM, contaminated equipment, etc. without proper labels.

Regulated Waste Disposal

All contaminated sharps shall be discarded as soon as feasible in sharps containers located in the facility. Sharps containers are located in: (specify locations of sharps containers).

Regulated waste other than sharps shall be placed in appropriate containers. Such containers are located in (specify locations of containers).

Laundry Procedures

Laundry contaminated with blood or other potentially infectious materials will be handled as little as possible. Such laundry will be placed in appropriately marked bags where it was used. Such laundry will not be sorted or rinsed in the area of use.

All employees who handle contaminated laundry will use personal protective equipment to prevent contact with blood or other potentially infectious materials.

Laundry at this facility will be cleaned at: _____ (specify location). (Employers should note here if the laundry is being sent off-site. If the laundry is being sent off-site, then the laundry service accepting the laundry is to be notified, in accordance with section (d) of the standard.)

Hepatitis B Vaccine

All employees who have been identified as having exposure to blood or other potentially infectious materials will be offered the Hepatitis B vaccine, at no cost to the employee. The vaccine will be offered within 10 working days of their initial assignment to work involving the potential for occupational exposure to blood or other potentially infectious materials unless the employee has previously had the vaccine or wishes to submit to antibody testing that shows the employee to have sufficient immunity.

Employees who decline the Hepatitis B vaccine will sign a waiver that uses the wording in Appendix A of the OSHA standard.

Employees who initially decline the vaccine but who later wish to have it while still covered under standard may then have the vaccine provided at no cost. (Employers should list here who has responsibility for assuring that the vaccine is offered, the waivers are signed, etc. Also the employer should list who will administer the vaccine.)

Documentation of refusal of the vaccination is kept at **(List location or person responsible for this recordkeeping).**

Vaccination will be provided by **(List Health Care Professional who is responsible for this part of the plan)** at **(location)** .

Following hepatitis B vaccinations, the health care professional's Written Opinion will be limited to whether the employee requires the hepatitis vaccine, and whether the vaccine was administered.

Post-Exposure Evaluation and Follow-Up

When the employee incurs an exposure incident, it should be reported to: (list who has responsibility to maintain records of exposure incident).

All employees who incur an exposure incident will be offered post-exposure evaluation and follow-up in accordance with the OSHA standard.

This follow-up will include the following:

- Documentation of the route of exposure and the circumstances related to the incident.

- If possible, the identification of the source individual and, if possible, the status of the source individual. The blood of the source individual will be tested (after consent is obtained for HIV/HBV infectivity).

- Results of testing of the source individual will be made available to the exposed employee with the exposed employee informed about the applicable laws and regulations concerning disclosure of the identity and infectivity of the source individual. (Employers may need to modify this provision in accordance with applicable local laws on this subject. Modifications should be listed here.)

- The employee will be offered the option of having their blood collected for testing of the employee's HIV/HBV serological status. The blood sample will be preserved for up to 90 days to allow the employee to decide if the blood should be tested for HIV serological status. However, if the employee decides before that time that testing will or will not be conducted then the appropriate action can be taken and the blood sample discarded.

- The employee will be offered post-exposure prophylaxis in accordance with the current recommendations of the U.S. Public Health Service. These recommendations are currently as follows: (these recommendations may be listed as an appendix to the plan).

- The employee will be given appropriate counseling concerning precautions to take during the period after the exposure incident. The employee will also be given information on what potential illness to be alert for and to report any related experiences to appropriate personnel.

The following person(s) has been designated to assure that the policy outlined here is effectively carried out as well as to maintain records related to this policy:

_____

Interaction with Health Care Professionals

A written opinion shall be obtained from the health care professional who evaluates employees of this facility. Written opinions will be obtained in the following instances:

1. When the employee is sent to obtain the Hepatitis B vaccine.

2. Whenever the employee is sent to a health care professional following an exposure incident.

3. Health care professionals shall be instructed to limit their opinions to:

4. Whether the Hepatitis B vaccine is indicated and if the employee has received the vaccine, or for evaluation following an incident.

5. That the employee has been informed of the results of the evaluation.

6. That the employee has been told about any medical conditions resulting from exposure to blood or other potentially infectious materials. (Note that the written opinion to the employer is not to reference any personal medical information.)

Employee Training

All employees who have occupational exposure to bloodborne pathogens receive training conducted by **(Name of responsible person or department). (Attach a brief description of their qualifications.)**

All employees who have occupational exposure to bloodborne pathogens receive training on the epidemiology, symptoms, and transmission of bloodborne pathogen diseases. In addition, the training program covers, at a minimum, the following elements:

1. a copy and explanation of the standard

2. an explanation of our ECP and how to obtain a copy

3. an explanation of methods to recognize tasks and other activities that may involve exposure to blood and OPIM, including what constitutes an exposure incident

4. an explanation of the use and limitations of engineering controls, work practices, and PPE

5. an explanation of the types, uses, location, removal, handling, decontamination, and disposal of PPE

6. an explanation of the basis for PPE selection

7. information on the hepatitis B vaccine, including information on its efficacy, safety, method of administration, the benefits of being vaccinated, and that the vaccine will be offered free of charge

8. information on the appropriate actions to take and persons to contact in an emergency involving blood or OPIM

9. an explanation of the procedure to follow if an exposure incident occurs, including the method of reporting the incident and the medical follow-up that will be made available

10. information on the post-exposure evaluation and follow-up that the employer is required to provide for the employee following an exposure incident

11. an explanation of the signs and labels and/or color coding required by the standard and used at this facility

12. an opportunity for interactive questions and answers with the person conducting the training session.

Training materials for this facility are available at

_____ .

Recordkeeping

Training Records

Training records are completed for each employee upon completion of training. These documents will be kept for at least **three years** at **(Name of responsible person or location of records)**.

The training records include:

- the dates of the training sessions

- the contents or a summary of the training sessions

- the names and qualifications of persons conducting the training

- the names and job titles of all persons attending the training sessions

Employee training records are provided upon request to the employee or the employee's authorized representative within 15 working days. Such requests should be addressed to **(Name of Responsible person or department)**.

Medical Records

Medical records are maintained for each employee with occupational exposure in accordance with 29 CFR 1910.20, "Access to Employee Exposure and Medical Records."

(Name of Responsible person or department) is responsible for maintenance of the required medical records. These **confidential** records are kept at **(List location)** for at least the **duration of employment plus 30 years.**

Employee medical records are provided upon request of the employee or to anyone having written consent of the employee within 15 working days. Such requests should be sent to **(Name of responsible person or department and address)**.

OSHA Recordkeeping

An exposure incident is evaluated to determine if the case meets OSHA's Recordkeeping Requirements (29 CFR 1904). This determination and the recording activities are done by **(Name of responsible person or department)**.

Appendix D

Tuberculosis (TB)

Introduction

Why Is Tuberculosis Included in a Bloodborne Pathogens Manual?

This section contains information about tuberculosis (TB), an airborne disease. Since 1985, the incidence of TB in the general U.S. population has increased approximately 14 percent, reversing a 30-year downward trend. Recently, drug-resistant strains of mycobacterium tuberculosis (M. tuberculosis) have become a serious concern and cases of multi-drug-resistant (MDR) TB have occurred in forty states. This overview of the risks of tuberculosis exposure (although it is not a bloodborne pathogen) has been added because many employees with occupational exposure to bloodborne pathogens may potentially have occupational exposure to persons with TB disease.

Nationwide, at least several hundred health care workers (HCW) have become infected with TB and have required medical treatment after workplace exposure to TB. Twelve (12) of these HCWs have died from TB disease. In general, persons who become infected with TB have approximately a 10-percent risk for developing TB disease in their lifetimes.

1994 CDC TB Guidelines

The Occupational Safety and Health Administration (OSHA) has not released a standard specific to tuberculosis (as of this printing); however, the Centers for Disease Control and Prevention (CDC) has released the 1994 TB Guidelines for the protection of HCWs. OSHA believes the CDC's 1994 TB Guidelines reflect an industry recognition of the hazard as well as appropriate, widely recognized, and accepted standards of practice to be followed by employers in carrying out their responsibilities under the Act.

The CDC is not a regulatory agency. The focus of the 1994 CDC TB Guidelines is to minimize the number of HCWs exposed to M. tuberculosis, while maintaining optimum care of patients with active infection with M. tuberculosis. The guidelines can be found in the "Morbidity and Mortality Weekly Report," vol. 43, October 28, 1994. No. RR-13 Recommendations and Reports: Guidelines for Preventing the Transmission of Mycobacterium Tuberculosis in Health-Care Facilities.

Occupational Safety and Health Act of 1970

OSHA is a regulatory agency. OSHA regulations are written to protect the employee from recognized hazards in the workplace. OSHA can and does enforce the worker protection by invoking the Occupational Safety and Health Act of 1970, or the General Duty Clause. The General Duty Clause (Public Law 91-596) states that "each employer shall furnish to each of his employees employment and a place of employment which are free from recognized hazards that are causing or are likely to cause death or serious physical harm to his employees: shall comply with occupational safety and health standards promulgated under this Act. Each employee shall comply with occupational safety and health standards and all rules, regulations, and orders issued pursuant to this Act which are applicable to his own actions and conduct."

Methods are available to minimize the hazards posed by employee exposure to TB. It is the employer's responsibility to see that these protections are in place and are readily available. It is your (the employee's) responsibility to utilize these protections.

Who Needs This Section?

Any employee who has potential for occupational exposure to M. tuberculosis needs this section. The 1994 CDC TB Guidelines specify five potentially hazardous work areas.

Healthcare facilities

Long-term care facilities for the elderly

Homeless shelters

Drug and treatment centers

Correctional facilities

The following is a list of HCWs whose tasks may lead them to occupational exposure to M. tuberculosis. The potential for occupational exposure is not limited to employees in these positions.

Physicians

Nurses

Aides

Home healthcare workers

Dental workers

Technicians

Workers in laboratories and morgues

Emergency medical service personnel

Students

Part-time personnel

Temporary staff not employed by the health care facility

Persons not directly involved with patient care, but who are potentially at risk for occupational exposure to M. tuberculosis (e.g., air ventilation system workers)

Meeting the General Duty Clause

The 1994 CDC TB Guidelines specify steps to be taken in order to minimize exposure to M. tuberculosis. In order to ensure a safe working environment and meet the OSHA General Duty Clause requirements, employers should provide the following:

1. An assessment of the risk for transmission of M. tuberculosis in the particular work setting

2. A protocol for the early identification of individuals with active TB

3. Training and information to ensure employee knowledge of the method of TB transmission, its signs and symptoms, medical surveillance and therapy, and site-specific protocols, including the purpose and proper use of controls (Note: failure to provide respirator training is citable under OSHA's general industry standard on respirators)

4. Medical screening, including pre-placement evaluation; administration and interpretation of Mantoux skin tests

5. Evaluation and management of workers with positive skin tests or a history of positive skin tests who are exhibiting symptoms of TB, including work restrictions for infectious employees

6. AFB (acid-fast bacilli) isolation rooms for suspected or confirmed infectious TB patients. These AFB isolation rooms, and areas in which high-hazard procedures are performed, should be single-patient rooms with special ventilation characteristics that are properly installed, maintained, and evaluated to reduce the potential for airborne exposure to M. tuberculosis.

7. Institution of Exposure Controls specific to the workplace which include the following:

   • Administrative Controls are policies and procedures to reduce the risk of employee exposure to infectious sources of M. tuberculosis. An example is a protocol to ensure rapid detection of people who are likely to have an active case of TB.

   • Engineering Controls attempt to design safety into the tools and workspace organization. An example is High Efficiency Particulate Air (HEPA) filtration systems.

   • Personal Respiratory Protective Equipment is used by the employee to prevent exposure to potentially infectious air droplet nuclei, for example, a personal respirator.

Tuberculosis (TB)

What Is Tuberculosis?

• M. tuberculosis is the bacteria responsible for causing TB in humans.

• TB is a disease that primarily spreads from person to person through droplet nuclei suspended in the air.

• TB may cause disease in any organ of the body. The most commonly affected organ is the lung, and accounts for about 85 percent of all infection sites. Other sites may include lymph nodes, the central nervous system, kidneys, and the skeletal system.

• TB is a serious and often fatal disease if left untreated.

• Symptoms of TB include weight loss, weakness, fever, night sweats, coughing, chest pain, and coughing up blood.

• The prevalence of infection is much higher in the close contacts of TB patients than in the general population.

• There is a difference between TB infection (positive TB skin test) and TB disease.

Transmission

TB is spread from person to person in the form of droplet nuclei in the air. When a person with TB coughs, sings, or laughs, the droplet nuclei are released into the air. When another uninfected person repeatedly breathes in the droplet nuclei, there is a chance of their becoming infected with TB.

For an employee to develop TB infection, he or she must have close contact to a sufficient number of air droplet nuclei over a long period of time. The employee's health is also considered as contributing to the susceptibility for TB infection and the possible development of TB disease. Among the medical risk factors for developing TB are diabetes, gastrectomy (removal of the stomach), long-term corticosteroid use, immunosuppressive therapy, cancers and other malignancies, and HIV infection.

Symptoms

Symptoms of TB also occur in people with more common diseases such as a cold or flu. The difference is that the symptoms of TB disease last longer than those of a cold or flu and must be treated with prescription antibiotics. The usual symptoms of TB disease include cough, production of sputum, weight loss, loss of appetite, weakness, fever, night sweats, malaise, fatigue, and, occasionally, chest pain. Hemoptysis, the coughing up of blood, may also occur, but usually not until after a person has had TB disease for some time.

Diagnosis

TB disease is diagnosed when there is a positive AFB sputum smear, or when three successive early morning sputum specimens are cultured and there is growth of M. tuberculosis from at least one culture. When extra-pulmonary (not in the lungs) TB is being considered, it may also be diagnosed by culture techniques. The difference is that the specimen is cultured from the site where TB is considered the cause of the infection.

Prevention

The 1994 CDC TB Guidelines recommend a hierarchy of controls to minimize TB transmission. These strategies are used in combination to promote workplace safety and to provide the employee with maximum protection against occupational exposure to M. tuberculosis. Under these guidelines, the control of TB is to be accomplished through the early identification, isolation, and treatment of persons with TB; use of engineering and administrative procedures to reduce the risk of exposure; and through the use of respiratory protection. The CDC 1994 TB Guidelines also stress the importance of the following measures: (1) use of risk assessments for developing a written TB control plan; (2) TB screening programs for HCWs; (3) HCW training and education; and (4) evaluation of TB infection-control programs.

TB Screening

Who Should Receive TB Screening?

According to the 1994 CDC TB Guidelines, HCWs are at increased risk for TB infection and should be provided with TB skin testing. This testing must be provided at no cost to employees at risk of exposure. The general population of the United States is thought to be at low risk for TB and should not be routinely tested.

Frequency of Testing

The frequency of testing is determined by the number of active cases of TB within a worksite of the facility. HCWs should receive TB skin testing prior to work in an area at increased risk for active cases of TB. A two-step TB skin testing process should be used (see What Is the Booster Effect?). Testing should be repeated each year, or more frequently for an employee assigned to a high-risk worksite or after a known exposure to a person with active TB.

What Is the TB Skin Test?

The tuberculin skin test of choice is the Mantoux test, which uses an intradermal injection of purified protein derivative (PPD). There are three strengths of PPD available; intermediate-strength (5 tuberculin units) PPD is the standard test material.

A skin test is done by injecting a very small amount of PPD just under the skin (usually the forearm is used). A small bleb (bubble) will be raised. The bleb will disappear. The injection site is then checked for reaction by your clinician about 48 to 72 hours later. If you fail to have the injection site evaluated in 72 hours, and no induration (swelling) is present, the tuberculin skin test will need to be repeated.

What Types of Reactions Occur?

Induration, the hard and bumpy swelling at the injection site, is used for determining a reaction to the PPD. Interpretation of results are best understood when the general health and risk of exposure to active TB cases are considered in the assessment. The injection site may also be red, but that does not determine a reaction to the PPD, nor indicate a positive result. We recommend that the interpretation guidelines of the American Thoracic Society–CDC Advisory panel be used to assess the measured induration at the injection site.

What Does a Positive Result Mean?

A positive skin test means an infection with M. tuberculosis has occurred, but does not prove TB disease. Referral for further medical evaluation is required to determine a diagnosis of TB disease. People found to have TB disease must be provided effective treatments. These treatments would be provided to the employee by the employer if the illness was found to be work related.

Possible False Positive Results

Close contacts of a person with TB disease, who have had a negative reaction to the first skin test, should be re-tested about 10 weeks after the last exposure to the person with TB disease. The delay between tests should allow enough time for the body's immune system to respond to an infection with M. tuberculosis. A second test will result in a positive reaction at the injection site if an infection with M. tuberculosis has occurred.

Contraindications to TB Screening

If you have tested positive to the TB skin test in the past it is not recommended that you receive the test again. Also, pregnancy does not exclude a HCW from being tested. Many pregnant workers have been tested for TB without documented harm to the fetus. You should consult with your doctor if you are pregnant and have any questions about receiving a TB skin test.

Post-Exposure Reporting

What Determines an Occupational Exposure?

Occupational exposure to M. tuberculosis is defined as employees working in one of the five types of facilities whose workers have been identified by the CDC as having a higher incidence of TB than the general population, and whose employees have exposure defined as follows:

1. Potential exposure to the exhaled air of an individual with suspected or confirmed TB disease

2. Exposure to a high-hazard procedure performed on an individual with suspected or confirmed TB disease, which could generate potentially infectious airborne droplet nuclei

What Is the Booster Effect?

Sensitivity to the TB skin test may decrease over time, causing an initial skin test to be negative but at the same time stimulating or boosting the immune system's sensitivity to tuberculin, thereby producing a positive reaction the next time the test is given. When repeated skin testing is necessary, concern about the booster effect and the misinterpretation of skin test results can be avoided by using a two-step testing process. This is why your employer should require the two-step test as soon as you start employment. The two-step test helps to eliminate any confusion over whether an employee was infected at the worksite or was previously infected (see Recordkeeping).

Post-Exposure Evaluation and Testing

Recordkeeping

Records of employee exposure to TB, skin tests, and medical evaluations and treatment must be maintained by your employer.

Active tuberculosis disease is an illness that must be reported to public health officials. Every state has reporting requirements.

For OSHA Form 200 recordkeeping purposes, both tuberculosis infections (positive TB skin test) and tuberculosis disease are recordable. A positive skin test for tuberculosis, even on initial testing (except preassignment screening), is recordable on the OSHA 200 log because of the presumption of work-relatedness in these settings, unless there is clear documentation that an outside exposure occurred.

Requirements

TB Exposure Control Plan

Employers having employees with exposure to TB shall establish a written Exposure Control Plan designed to eliminate or minimize employee exposure. This plan involves:

· Schedule and method of implementation of the control plan

· PPD testing

· Respiratory protection

· Communication of hazards to employees

· Post-exposure evaluation and follow-up

· Recordkeeping

Relationship to HIV

1. People infected with HIV and M. tuberculosis are at a very high risk of developing active TB. Seven to 10 percent of persons infected with both TB and HIV will develop active disease each year.

2. Extrapulmonary TB (i.e., outside the lungs) is more common in people with HIV infections.

3. Miliary TB and lymphatic TB are more common in HIV-infected people.

4. The HIV epidemic is a major contributing factor to the recent increase in cases of active

Appendix E

OSHA Directory

U.S. Department of Labor Occupational Safety and Health Administration Regional Offices

Region I
(CT*, MA , ME, NH, RI, VT*)
133 Portland Street
1st Floor
Boston,MA 02114
Telephone: (617) 565-7164

Region II
(NJ, NY*, PR*, VI*)
201 Varick Street
Room 670
New York, NY 10014
Telephone: (212) 337-2378

Region III
(DC, DE, MD*, PA, VA, WV*)
Gateway Building, Suite 2100
3535 Market Street
Philadelphia, PA 19104
Telephone: (215) 596-1201

Region IV
(AL, FL, GA, KY*, MS, NC*, SC*, TN*)
1375 Peachtree Street, N.E.
Suite 587
Atlanta, GA 30367
Telephone: (404) 347-3573

Region V
(IL, IN*, MI*, MN*, OH, WI)
230 South Dearborn Street
Room 3244
Chicago, IL 60604
Telephone: (312) 353-2220

Region VI
(AR, LA, NM*, OK, TX)
525 Griffin Street
Room 602
Dallas, TX 75202
Telephone: (214) 767-4731

Region VII
(IA*, KS, MO, NE)
911 Walnut Street, Room 406
Kansas City, MO 64106
Telephone: (816) 426-5861

Region VIII
(CO, MT, ND, SD, UT*, WY*)
Federal Building, Room 1576
1961 Stout Street
Denver, CO 80294
Telephone: (303) 844-3061

Region IX
(Amercian Samoa, AZ*, CA*, Guam, HI*, NV*,
Trust Territories of the Pacific)
71 Stevenson Street
Room 415
San Francisco, CA 94105
Telephone: (415) 744-6670

Region X
(AK*, ID, OR*, WA*)
1111 Third Avenue
Suite 715
Seattle, WA 98101-3212
Telephone: (206) 553-5930

*These states and territories operate their own OSHA-approved job safety and health programs (Connecticut and New York plans cover public employees only). States with approved programs must have a standard that is identical to, or at least as effective as, the federal standard.

Appendix F

Answers to End of Chapter Learning Activities

Chapter One Answers

1. Drawing blood, transporting blood, housekeeping in a healthcare facility
2. True
3. True
4. True
5. Yes
6. construction, agriculture, marine terminal, or longshore industries
7. Yes
8. Yes
9. Yes

Chapter Two Answers

1. HBV
2. True
3. Jaundice, Fever
4. True
5. True
6. True
7. Yes
8. True
9. True
10. True
11. True
12. Yes
13. No
14. HIV
15. True

Chapter Three Answers

1. No
2. True
3. True
4. False
5. False
6. True

Glossary

A

AFB: Acid-fast bacilli.

AIDS: Acquired Immunodeficiency Syndrome, a disease that results from HIV.

airborne: Capable of being transmitted by air particles.

anorexia: Loss of appetite.

antigen: A substance that causes antibody formation.

B

biological cabinet: a device enclosed except for necessary exhaust purposes on three sides and top and bottom, designed to draw air inward by means of mechanical ventilation, operated with insertion of only the hands and arms of the user, and in which virulent pathogens are used. Biological cabinets are classified as Class I, Class II, and Class III.

blood: The term "human blood components" includes plasma, platelets, and serosanguinous fluids (e.g., exudates from wounds). Also included are medications derived from blood, such as immune globulins, albumin, and factors 8 and 9.

bloodborne pathogen: While HBV and HIV are specifically identified in the standard, the term includes any pathogenic microorganism that is present in human blood or OPIM and can infect and cause disease in persons who are exposed to blood containing the pathogen.

C

clinical laboratory: a workplace where diagnostic or other screening procedures are performed on blood or other potentially infectious materials.

contaminated: The presence or the reasonably anticipated presence of blood or other potentially infectious materials on an item or surface.

contaminated laundry: Laundry that has been soiled with blood or other potentially infectious materials or may contain sharps.

contaminated sharps: Any contaminated object that can penetrate the skin including, but not limited to, needles, scalpels, broken capillary tubes, and exposed ends of dental wires.

D

decontamination: The use of physical or chemical means to remove, inactivate, or destroy bloodborne pathogens on a surface or item to the point where they are no longer capable of transmitting infectious particles and the surface or item is rendered safe for handling, use, or disposal.

DeLee suctioning: An emergency method of clearing an infant's airway.

E

engineering controls: Physical controls (e.g., sharps disposal containers, self-sheathing needles, etc.) that isolate or remove the bloodborne pathogens hazard from the workplace.

Engineered Sharps Injury Protection: means either:

(1) A physical attribute built into a needle device used for withdrawing body fluids, accessing a vein or artery, or administering medications or other fluids, which effectively reduces the risk of an exposure incident by a mechanism such as barrier creation, blunting, encapsulation, withdrawal or other effective mechanisms; or

(2) A physical attribute built into any other type of needle device, or into a non-needle sharp, which effectively reduces the risk of an exposure incident.

exposure incident: A specific eye, mouth, other mucous membrane, non-intact skin, or parenteral contact with blood or other potentially infectious materials that results from the performance of an employee's duties.

extrapulmonary: Outside of the lungs.

H

handwashing facility: A facility that provides an adequate supply of running potable water, soap, and single use towels or hot air drying machines.

HBV: Hepatitis B Virus. One of the viruses that causes illness directly affecting the liver. It is a bloodborne pathogen.

HCV: is a viral infection of the liver that is transmitted primarily by exposure to blood. Currently there is no vaccine effective against HCV.

HEPA: High-efficiency particulate air filter.

hepatitis: A disease that causes swelling, soreness, and loss of normal function of the liver. Symptoms include weakness, fatigue, anorexia, nausea, abdominal pain, fever, and headache. Jaundice is a symptom that may develop later.

HIV: Human Immunodeficiency Virus is a virus that infects immune system blood cells in humans and renders them less effective in preventing disease.

I

immune: Resistant to infectious disease.

immunization: A process or procedure by which resistance to infectious disease is produced in a person.

J

jaundice: A yellowing of the skin associated with hepatitis infection.

L

Licensed Healthcare Professional: a person whose legally permitted licensed scope of practice allows includes him or her to independently perform the an activities required by subsection (f), Hepatitis B Vaccination and Post-exposure Evaluation and Follow-up which this section requires to be performed by a licensed healthcare professional.

M

mucous membrane: Any one of the four types of thin sheets of tissue that cover or line various parts of the body. An example would be the skin lining the nose and mouth.

mucus: The clear secretion of the mucous membrane.

N

needle: A needle of any type, including, but not limited to, solid and hollow-bore needles.

needleless system: A device that does not utilize needles for:

(1) The withdrawal of body fluids after initial venous or arterial access is established;

(2) The administration of medication or fluids; and

(3) Any other procedure involving the potential for an exposure incident.

NIOSH: The National Institute for Occupational Safety and Health, U.S. Department of Health and Human Services, or designated representative.

non-intact skin: Skin that has a break in the surface. It includes but is not limited to abrasions, cuts, hangnails, paper cuts, and burns.

nuclei: A particle that makes up a nucleus of an atom.

O

occupational: Job related.

occupational exposure: Reasonably anticipated skin, eye, mucous membrane, or parenteral contact with blood or other potentially infectious materials that may result from the performance of an employee's duties. "Reasonably anticipated contact" includes, among others, contact with blood or OPIM (including regulated waste) as well as incidents of needlesticks.

one-hand technique: A procedure wherein the needle of a reusable syringe is capped in a sterile manner during use. The technique employed shall require the use of only the hand holding the syringe so that the free hand is not exposed to the uncapped needle.

Other Potentially Infectious Materials (OPIM): Coverage under this definition also extends to blood and tissues of experimental animals who are infected with HIV or HBV.

P

parenteral: Piercing mucous membranes or the skin barrier through such events as needle sticks, human bites, cuts, and abrasion.

pathogen: Any virus, microorganism, or other substance that is capable of causing disease.

percutaneous: Performed through the skin as in draining fluid from an abscess using a needle.

personal protective equipment: Specialized clothing or equipment worn or used by an employee for protection against a hazard. General work clothes (e.g., uniforms, pants, shirts or blouses) not intended to function as protection against a hazard are not considered to be personal protective equipment.

production facility: a facility engaged in industrial-scale, large-volume or high concentration production of HIV, or HBV or HCV.

R

regulated waste: liquid or semi-liquid blood or other potentially infectious materials; contaminated items that would release blood or other potentially infectious materials in a liquid or semi-liquid state if compressed; items that are caked with dried blood or other potentially infectious materials and are capable of releasing these materials during handling; contaminated sharps; and pathological and microbiological wastes containing blood or other potentially infectious materials.

research laboratory: a laboratory producing or using research-laboratory-scale amounts of HIV, or HBV or HCV. Research laboratories may produce high concentrations of HIV, or HBV or HCV but not in the volume found in production facilities.

respirator: A mechanical device used to assist breathing. In this case it refers to a device used to filter particles from the air.

S

sharp: any object used or encountered in the industries covered by subsection (a) that can be reasonably anticipated to penetrate the skin or any other part of the body, and to result in an exposure incident, including, but not limited to, needle devices, scalpels, lancets, broken glass, broken capillary tubes, exposed ends of dental wires and dental knives, drills and burs.

sharps injury: any injury caused by a sharp, including, but not limited to, cuts, abrasions, or needlesticks.

sharps injury log: a written or electronic record satisfying the requirements of subsection (c)(2).

source individual: Any individual, living or dead, whose blood or other potentially infectious materials may be a source of occupational exposure to the employee. Examples include, but are not limited to, hospital and clinic patients; clients in institutions for the developmentally disabled; trauma victims; clients of drug and alcohol treatment facilities; residents of hospices and nursing homes; human remains; and individuals who donate or sell blood or blood components.

sterilize: The use of a physical or chemical procedure to destroy all microbial life including highly resistant bacterial endospores.

T

T4: A cell in the immune system that acts as a sensor to activate the immune system.

TB disease: Having the organism that causes TB in the body, in its active state. A person with TB disease usually has symptoms and can transmit the disease to others.

TB infection: Having the organism that causes TB in the body, but not having the active disease. A person having TB infection is asymptomatic and cannot transmit TB unless the organism converts to an active state.

U

Universal Precautions: an approach to infection control. According to the concept of Universal Precautions, all human blood and certain human body fluids are treated as if known to be infectious for HIV, HBV, HCV, and other bloodborne pathogens.

V

vaccine: A suspension of inactive or killed microorganisms administered orally or injected into a human to induce active immunity to infectious disease.

W

work practice controls: controls that reduce the likelihood of exposure by altering defining the manner in which a task is performed (e.g., prohibiting recapping of needles by a two-handed technique and use of patient-handling techniques).

Quick Emergency Index